Cooking for Type 2-Diabetes; Satisfying and Nutrient-Rich Meals

Clara Barton B.

This book highlights its focus on nutritious yet delightful meals, and its practical tips for those managing Type 2 Diabetes. It invites readers to embark on a culinary journey that supports their health and culinary pleasure.

Contents

Figuring out Type 2 Diabetes

NO-TO-TYPE 2-DIABETES

The cookbook gives far reaching data about type 2 diabetes, including its causes, side effects, and the executives techniques. Perusers can acquire a superior comprehension of their condition.

Dietary Direction: The cookbook offers viable direction on keeping a fair eating routine, which is significant for overseeing glucose levels. Perusers can figure out how to settle on better food decisions and make adjusted feasts.

Recipe Assortment: The cookbook includes a different scope of recipes, from breakfast to treat and in the middle between. Perusers can get close enough to tasty and diabetes-accommodating recipes that make dinner arranging simpler and more charming.

Cooking Tips

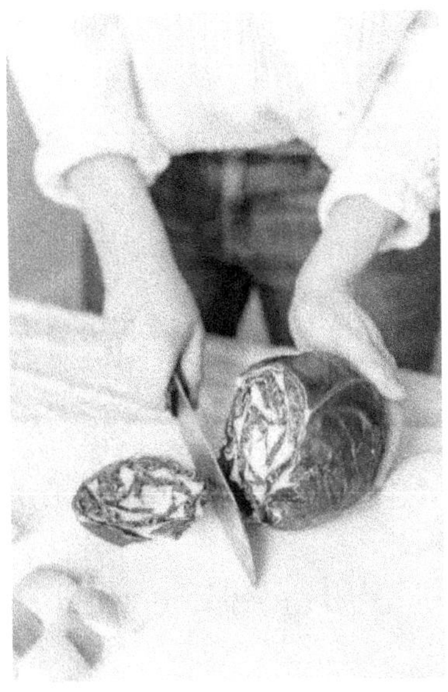

The cookbook incorporates cooking tips and strategies that assist per users with planning dinners that are nutritious as well as tasty. These tips can improve cooking abilities and trust in the kitchen.

Segment Control: Perusers can find out about the significance of part control and how to apply it in their everyday dinners. This information can support better piece the executives and further developed glucose control.

Fixing Replacements: The cookbook offers data on fixing replacements, permitting perusers to settle on better decisions while as yet getting a charge out of delicious dishes. This is especially useful for decreasing sugar and unfortunate fats in recipes.

Feast Arranging Methodologies: Perusers can acquire bits of knowledge into successful dinner arranging techniques, which can work on shopping for food, save time in the kitchen, and backing reliable glucose the board.

Smart dieting Propensities: By following the cookbook's proposals and recipes, perusers can develop good dieting propensities that advance generally prosperity, not simply diabetes the executives.

Assortment in Dinners: The cookbook gives a wide assortment of recipes, guaranteeing that perusers can appreciate different and fulfilling feasts without feeling limited.

Assets and References: The supplements of the cookbook offer extra assets, including a glossary of cooking terms, a rundown of normal fixings, and connections to additional data and backing.

Perusers can involve these assets for continuous learning and help.

Record: The file permits perusers to rapidly track down unambiguous recipes, tips, and data inside the cookbook, making it a convenient reference instrument.

Trust in Cooking: With the direction and recipes gave, perusers can acquire trust in their capacity to plan heavenly and diabetes-accommodating dinners, prompting more prominent freedom in dealing with their condition.

Further developed Wellbeing: At last, perusers can acquire further developed wellbeing results by following the cookbook's suggestions and recipes.

Better glucose control, weight the board, and generally prosperity are among the expected advantages.

Delight in Food: Significantly, perusers can keep on partaking in the joys of food and preparing while at the same time overseeing type 2 diabetes. The cookbook underscores that delectable feasts can be important for a reasonable and healthy way of life.

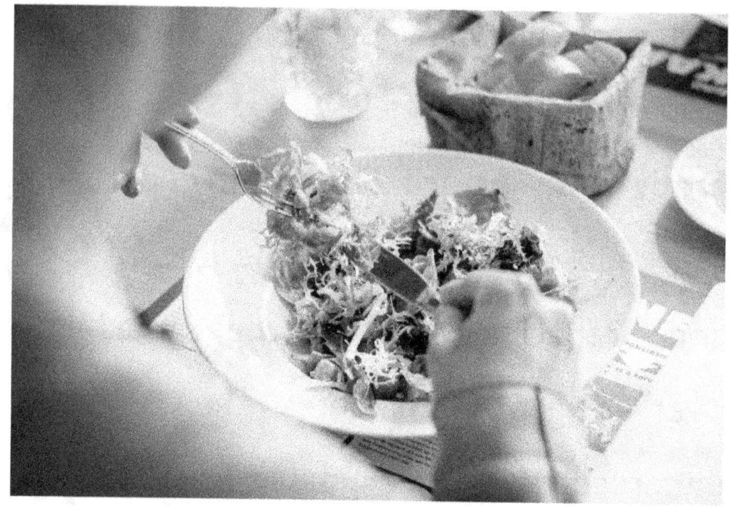

Eating great with type 2 diabetes is fundamental for overseeing glucose levels and generally speaking wellbeing. Here are a few key standards:

Balanced Diet: Hold back nothing balanced diet wealthy in vegetables, organic products, entire grains, lean proteins, and solid fats. This gives fundamental supplements and balance out glucose.

Carbohydrate Management: Screen carbohydrate consumption, as carbs fundamentally influence glucose levels. Pick complex starches like entire grains and vegetables over refined carbs.

Segment Control: Be aware of part sizes to abstain from indulging. Controlling bits oversees calorie admission and glucose levels.

Fiber-Rich Food varieties: Integrate fiber-rich food sources like beans, lentils, vegetables, and entire grains. Fiber dials back the retention of glucose, advancing better glucose control.

Limit Sugary and Handled Food sources: Diminish or take out sugary refreshments, desserts, and vigorously handled food varieties. These can cause quick spikes in glucose.

Healthy Fats: Incorporate wellsprings of healthy fats, like avocados, nuts, seeds, and olive oil, while restricting immersed and trans fats.

Ordinary Feasts: Eat at customary spans to keep up with stable glucose levels. Skipping feasts can prompt glucose changes.

Observing: Routinely screen your glucose levels as suggested by your medical services supplier. This evaluates the effect of various food varieties on your body.

Coordinated effort: Work with an enrolled dietitian or nutritionist spend significant time in diabetes the executives to make a customized feast plan.

Kitchen Tips for Healthy Cooking:

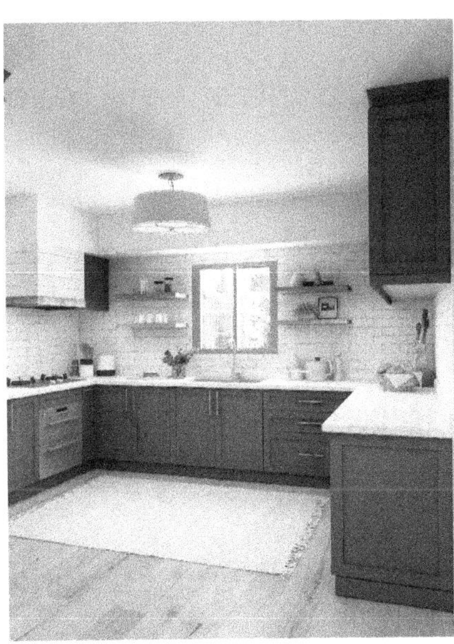

Making a diabetes-accommodating kitchen and embracing solid cooking practices can make it simpler to keep a fair eating regimen. Here are some kitchen tips:

Stocking Healthy Food Stuffs: Keep your storeroom and cooler supplied with healthy fixings like entire grains, lean proteins, new produce, and low-sodium canned products.

Meal Arranging: Plan your feasts and snacks early on to guarantee you have adjusted choices accessible.

Diminishing Sugars: Supplant sugar in recipes with sugar substitutes or lessen how much sugar utilized in cooking and baking.

Cooking Strategies: Pick better cooking techniques like barbecuing, baking, steaming, and sautéing, which require less oil than broiling.

Segment Control: Use estimating cups and kitchen scales to control segment measures and abstain from indulging.

Flavor Enhancers: Use spices, flavors, and citrus natural products to add flavor to dishes without depending on overabundance salt or sugar.

Mark Perusing: Read food names to check for buried sugars, over the top sodium, and undesirable fats in bundled food varieties.

Testing: Investigate new recipes and fixings that line up with your dietary objectives, making smart dieting seriously energizing.

Remain Coordinated: Keep your kitchen coordinated and liberated from mess to make feast planning more effective.

Breakfast Recipes

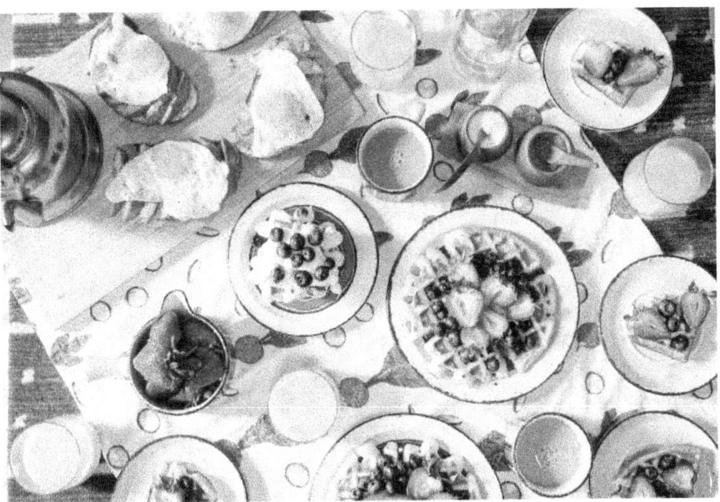

The first meal of the day, breakfast is often eaten in the morning. In English, the phrase refers to breaking the previous night's fast. In the short term, it boosts your energy and concentration, while in the long run, it can help you better manage your weight and lower your chances of developing heart disease and type 2 diabetes.

Hearty Oatmeal with Berries

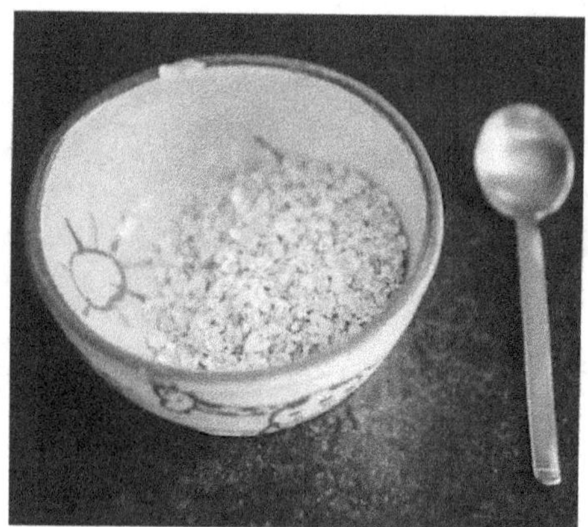

Ingredients:

- 1/2 cup rolled oats
- 1 cup almond milk (or any milk of your choice)
- 1/4 teaspoon cinnamon
- 1/4 cup mixed berries (strawberries, blueberries, raspberries)
- 1 tablespoon chopped nuts (almonds, walnuts, or pecans)
- 1 teaspoon honey or maple syrup (optional for sweetness)

Instructions:

- In a small saucepan, combine the rolled oats and almond milk.
- Bring the mixture to a boil over medium heat, stirring occasionally.
- Reduce the heat to low and add the cinnamon. Simmer for about 5 minutes, or until the oats are creamy and cooked to your liking.
- Remove from heat and transfer the oatmeal to a bowl.
- Top with mixed berries, chopped nuts, and a drizzle of honey or maple syrup, if desired.
- Serve hot and enjoy your hearty oatmeal with berries!

Veggie and Cheese Omelette

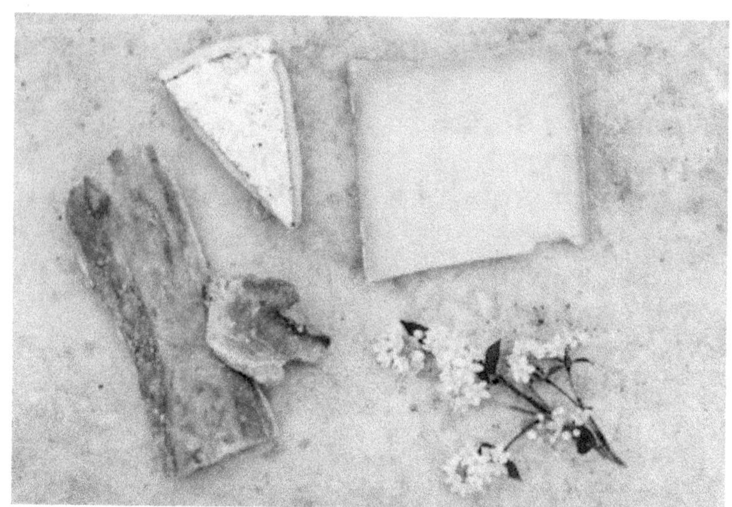

Ingredients:

+ 2 large eggs

+ 2 tablespoons diced bell peppers (red, green, or yellow)

+ 2 tablespoons diced onions

+ 2 tablespoons diced tomatoes

+ 2 tablespoons shredded low-fat cheese (cheddar, mozzarella, or your choice)

+ Salt and pepper to taste

+ Cooking spray or a small amount of olive oil for the pan

Instructions:

+ In a bowl, whisk the eggs until well beaten. Season with a pinch of salt and pepper.

+ Heat a non-stick skillet over medium heat and lightly coat it with cooking spray or a small amount of olive oil.

+ Add the diced bell peppers and onions to the skillet and sauté for 2-3 minutes until they start to soften.

- Pour the beaten eggs into the skillet, swirling them around to evenly distribute the vegetables.

- As the edges of the omelette begin to set, use a spatula to gently lift the edges and tilt the pan to let the uncooked egg flow underneath.

- Once the omelette is mostly set but still slightly runny on top, sprinkle the diced tomatoes and shredded cheese evenly over one half of the omelette.

- Carefully fold the other half of the omelette over the cheese and tomatoes to create a half-moon shape.

- Cook for another minute or until the cheese has melted, and the omelette is fully cooked.
- Slide the omelette onto a plate, cut in half, and serve hot.

Greek Yogurt Parfait

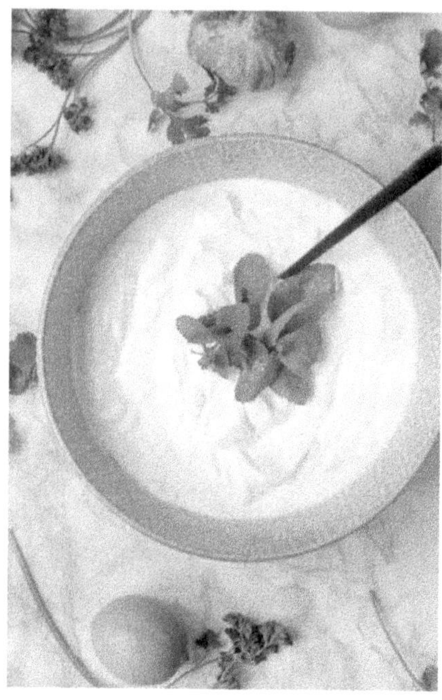

Ingredients:

+ 1/2 cup Greek yogurt (plain or flavored)
+ 1/4 cup granola (choose a low-sugar option)
+ 1/4 cup mixed berries (strawberries, blueberries, raspberries)
+ 1 tablespoon honey (optional for sweetness)

Instructions:

- In a glass or bowl, layer half of the Greek yogurt.
- Add half of the granola on top of the yogurt layer.
- Layer half of the mixed berries on top of the granola.
- Repeat the layers with the remaining yogurt, granola, and berries.
- Drizzle honey over the top if you desire extra sweetness.
- Serve immediately and enjoy your Greek yogurt parfait!

Whole Grain Pancakes

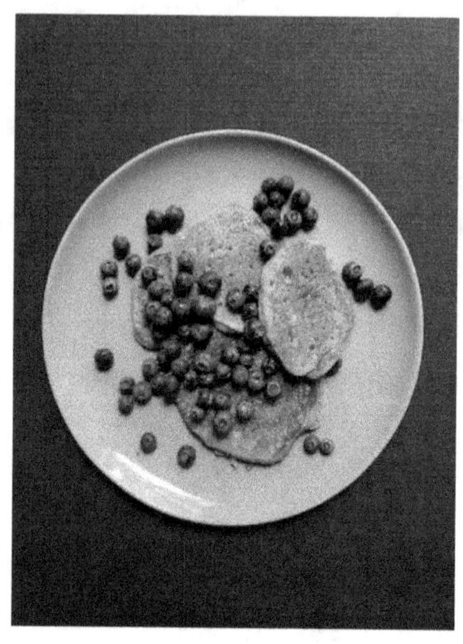

Ingredients:

- 1 cup whole wheat flour
- 1 tablespoon sugar or a sugar substitute
- 1 teaspoon baking powder
- 1/2 teaspoon baking soda
- 1/4 teaspoon salt
- 1 cup buttermilk or a milk alternative
- 1 large egg
- 1 tablespoon melted butter or vegetable oil

+ Cooking spray or a small amount of butter for the pan

Instructions:

+ In a mixing bowl, whisk together the whole wheat flour, sugar (or sugar substitute), baking powder, baking soda, and salt.
+ In another bowl, beat the egg and then add the buttermilk and melted butter (or oil).
+ Pour the wet ingredients into the dry ingredients and stir until just combined. Do not overmix; it's okay if there are some lumps.

- Heat a non-stick skillet or griddle over medium heat and lightly coat it with cooking spray or butter.
- Pour 1/4 cup portions of batter onto the skillet to make individual pancakes.
- Cook until bubbles form on the surface, then flip the pancakes and cook the other side until golden brown.
- Remove the pancakes from the skillet and keep warm.
- Serve with your choice of toppings, such as fresh berries, a dollop of Greek yogurt, or a drizzle of maple syrup.

Avocado Toast with Poached Eggs

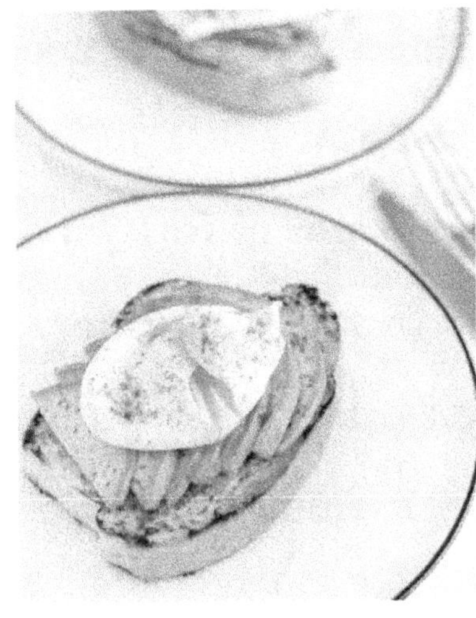

Ingredients:

+ 2 slices of whole grain bread
+ 1 ripe avocado
+ 2 large eggs
+ Salt and pepper to taste
+ Optional toppings: diced tomatoes, red pepper flakes, or a sprinkle of grated Parmesan cheese

Instructions:

+ Toast the slices of whole grain bread to your desired level of crispness.

- While the bread is toasting, cut the ripe avocado in half, remove the pit, and scoop the flesh into a bowl.
- Mash the avocado with a fork and season with a pinch of salt and pepper.
- In a saucepan, bring water to a gentle simmer (not boiling). Add a splash of vinegar if desired; it helps the eggs hold their shape while poaching.
- Crack one egg into a small bowl or ramekin.
- Create a gentle whirlpool in the simmering water with a spoon and carefully slide the egg into the center of the whirlpool. This helps the egg white wrap around the yolk.

- Poach the egg for about 3-4 minutes for a runny yolk or longer for a firmer yolk.
- Use a slotted spoon to remove the poached egg from the water and drain any excess water.
- Repeat the poaching process with the second egg.
- Spread the mashed avocado evenly onto the toasted bread slices.
- Place a poached egg on top of each avocado toast.
- Season with additional salt, pepper, and your choice of toppings.
- Serve immediately, and enjoy your avocado toast with poached eggs!

Appetizers and Snacks

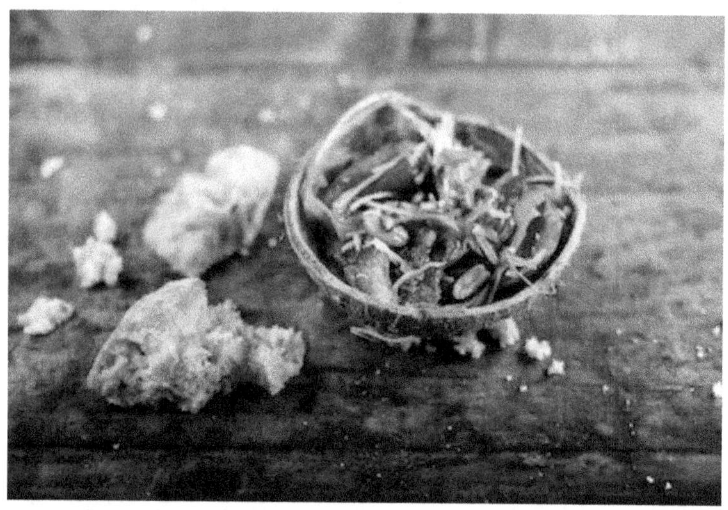

An appetizer is a small serving of food that is served before the main meal with the goal of piqueing the diner's interest in what is to come. A snack is a small meal consumed in between meals, or occasionally in place of a meal, with the goal of satiating hunger until a larger meal is available.

Roasted Red Pepper Hummus

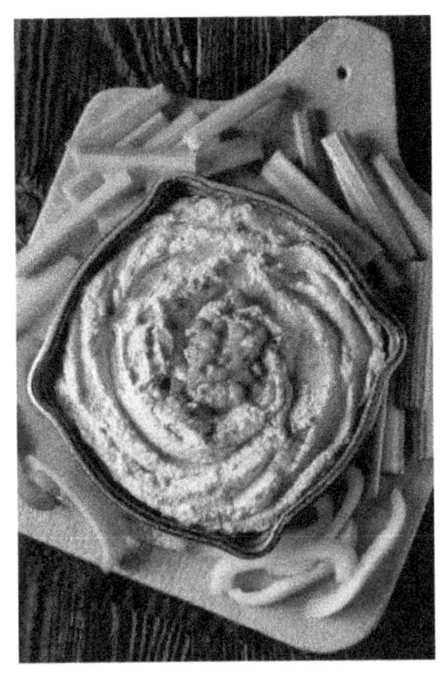

<u>Ingredients:</u>

- 1 (15-ounce) can chickpeas (garbanzo beans), drained and rinsed
- 1/3 cup roasted red pepper strips (from a jar or homemade)
- 2 tablespoons tahini (sesame paste)
- 2 cloves garlic, minced
- 2 tablespoons fresh lemon juice
- 2 tablespoons olive oil
- 1/2 teaspoon ground cumin
- Salt and pepper to taste

➕ Optional garnish: chopped fresh parsley,
a drizzle of olive oil

Instructions:

➕ In a food processor, combine the chickpeas, roasted red pepper strips, tahini, minced garlic, lemon juice, olive oil, and ground cumin.

➕ Process the ingredients until smooth, pausing to scrape down the sides of the bowl as needed.

➕ If the hummus is too thick, you can add a bit of water (1-2 tablespoons) to achieve the desired consistency.

➕ Season with salt and pepper to taste, and pulse to combine.

+ Transfer the roasted red pepper hummus to a serving bowl.

+ Drizzle with a bit of olive oil and sprinkle with chopped fresh parsley if desired.

+ Serve with pita bread, fresh vegetables, or whole-grain crackers for dipping.

Cucumber and Tomato Salad

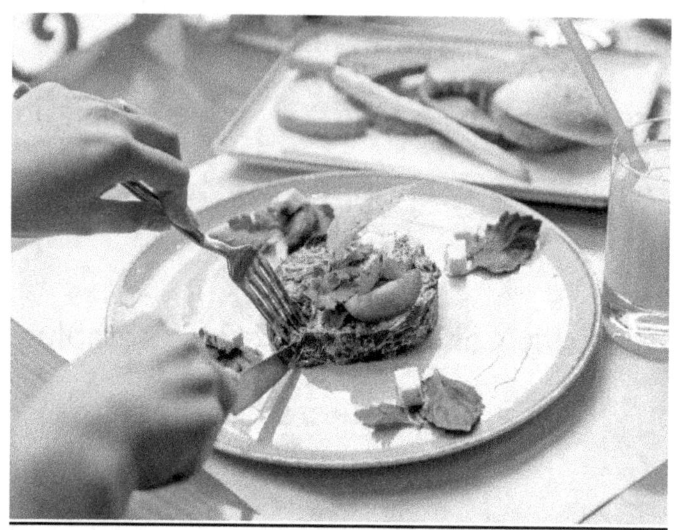

Ingredients:

- 2 cucumbers, peeled and sliced
- 2 large tomatoes, diced
- 1/2 red onion, thinly sliced
- 1/4 cup fresh parsley, chopped
- 2 tablespoons extra-virgin olive oil
- 2 tablespoons red wine vinegar
- Salt and pepper to taste

Instructions:

- In a large bowl, combine the cucumber slices, diced tomatoes, sliced red onion, and chopped parsley.
- In a small bowl, whisk together the extra-virgin olive oil and red wine vinegar to make the dressing.
- Drizzle the dressing over the cucumber and tomato mixture.
- Season with salt and pepper to taste.
- Toss the salad gently to combine all the ingredients and coat them with the dressing.
- Refrigerate for about 15-30 minutes before serving to allow the flavors to meld.

+ Serve chilled as a refreshing snack or appetizer.

Baked Sweet Potato Fries

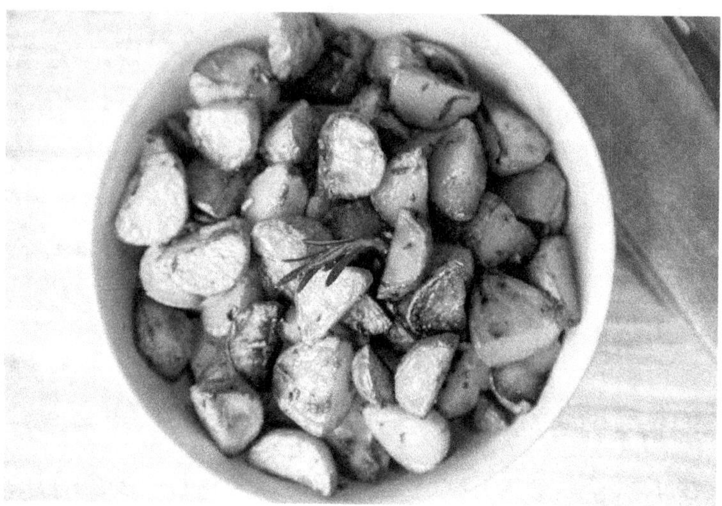

<u>Ingredients:</u>

+ 2 medium sweet potatoes, peeled and cut into fries

+ 2 tablespoons olive oil

+ 1/2 teaspoon paprika

* 1/2 teaspoon garlic powder

* 1/4 teaspoon salt

* 1/4 teaspoon black pepper

* Cooking spray (for the baking sheet)

Instructions:

* Preheat your oven to 425°F (220°C) and line a baking sheet with aluminum foil. Lightly coat the foil with cooking spray to prevent sticking.

* In a large bowl, toss the sweet potato fries with olive oil, paprika, garlic powder, salt, and black pepper until they are evenly coated.

* Arrange the seasoned sweet potato fries in a single layer on the prepared

baking sheet, ensuring they are not crowded.

+ Bake in the preheated oven for 20-25 minutes, flipping the fries halfway through, or until they are crispy and golden brown.

+ Remove from the oven and let cool slightly before serving.

+ Enjoy your baked sweet potato fries as a healthier alternative to traditional fries!

Guacamole with Whole Wheat Pita

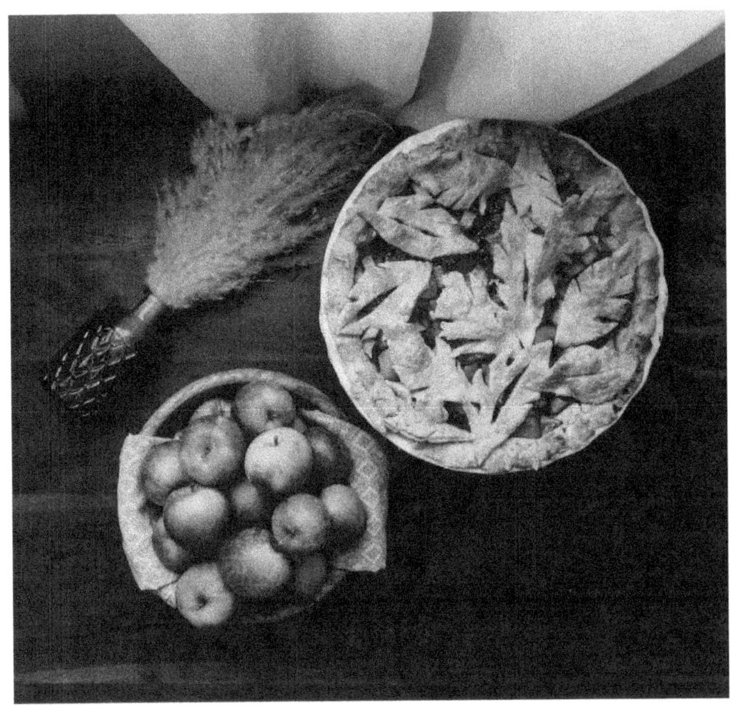

Ingredients:

- 2 ripe avocados, peeled and pitted
- 1 small tomato, diced
- 1/4 cup red onion, finely chopped
- 1 clove garlic, minced

+ 2 tablespoons fresh lime juice

+ 1/4 teaspoon salt

+ 1/4 teaspoon ground cumin

+ 1/4 teaspoon chili powder

+ 2 whole wheat pita bread, cut into triangles (for serving)

Instructions:

+ In a bowl, mash the ripe avocados with a fork until smooth, leaving some chunks for texture.

+ Add the diced tomato, finely chopped red onion, minced garlic, fresh lime juice, salt, ground cumin, and chili powder to the mashed avocado. Stir to combine all the ingredients thoroughly.

+ Taste the guacamole and adjust the seasonings, if needed, by adding more salt or lime juice.

+ Serve the guacamole with whole wheat pita bread triangles for dipping.

+ Enjoy this nutritious and flavorful snack!

Spiced Nuts

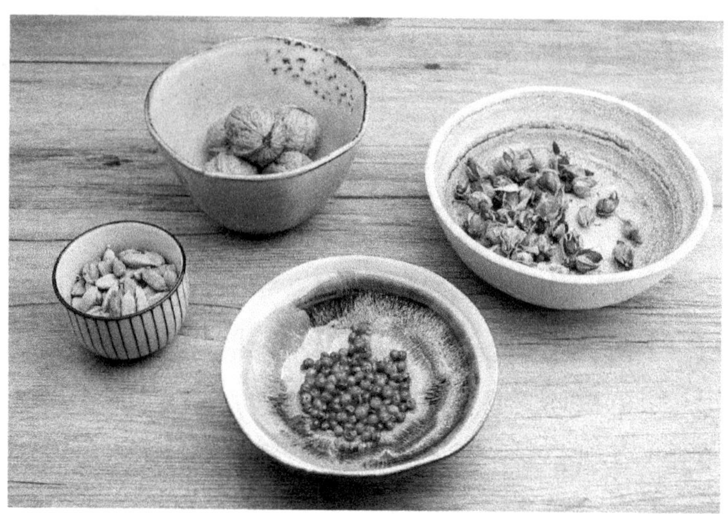

Ingredients:

- 2 cups mixed nuts (such as almonds, walnuts, and cashews)
- 1 egg white
- 1 tablespoon water
- 1/4 cup granulated sugar or a sugar substitute
- 1 teaspoon ground cinnamon

- 1/4 teaspoon ground cayenne pepper (adjust to taste for spiciness)
- 1/4 teaspoon salt

Instructions:

- Preheat your oven to 300°F (150°C). Line a baking sheet with parchment paper.
- In a bowl, whisk together the egg white and water until frothy.
- Add the mixed nuts to the egg white mixture and stir to coat evenly.
- In a separate bowl, mix the granulated sugar (or sugar substitute), ground cinnamon, ground cayenne pepper, and salt.

- Sprinkle the spice mixture over the coated nuts and toss to ensure all the nuts are well coated.
- Spread the spiced nuts evenly on the prepared baking sheet.
- Bake in the preheated oven for about 25-30 minutes, stirring every 10 minutes, until the nuts are golden brown and fragrant.
- Remove from the oven and let cool completely. The nuts will become crisp as they cool.
- Once cooled, store the spiced nuts in an airtight container.
- Enjoy these savory and slightly spicy nuts as a delightful snack!

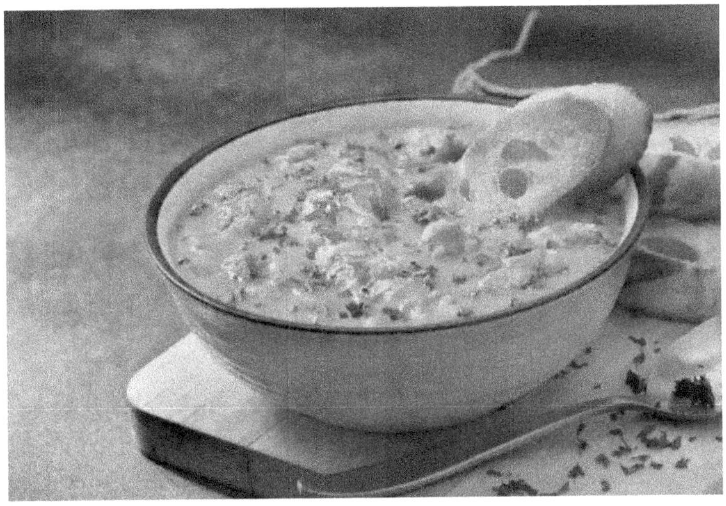

Soup is a type of liquid cuisine that frequently includes chunks of solid food and has a base of meat, fish, or vegetables.

While

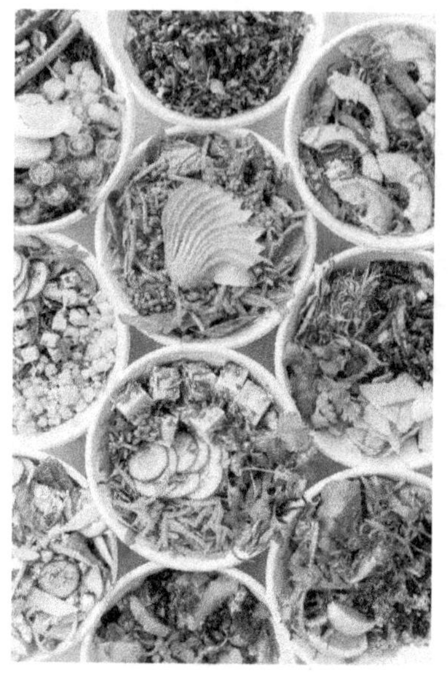 Salads is a combination of raw vegetables, typically comprising lettuce, that is consumed alone or with additional foods: Mix the vinaigrette dressing into the salad before tossing. Serve a fresh salad beside the risotto. a salad that is made with cheese, tuna, eggs, etc.

Minestrone Soup

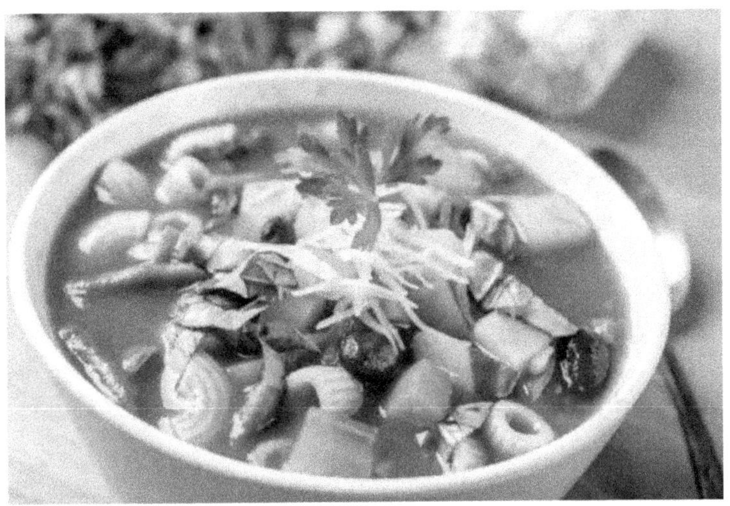

Ingredients:

- 1 tablespoon olive oil
- 1 small onion, diced
- 2 cloves garlic, minced
- 1 medium carrot, diced
- 1 celery stalk, diced
- 1 zucchini, diced
- 1 cup green beans, chopped

- 1 (14.5-ounce) can diced tomatoes
- 1 (15-ounce) can kidney beans, drained and rinsed
- 1/2 cup small pasta (e.g., small shells or elbow macaroni)
- 6 cups vegetable broth (low-sodium)
- 1 teaspoon dried basil
- 1 teaspoon dried oregano
- Salt and pepper to taste
- Grated Parmesan cheese (optional for garnish)
- Fresh basil leaves (optional for garnish)

Instructions:

- In a large soup pot, heat the olive oil over medium heat.

- Add the diced onion, minced garlic, diced carrot, and diced celery. Sauté for about 5 minutes, or until the vegetables begin to soften.
- Add the diced zucchini and chopped green beans to the pot and continue to cook for another 3-4 minutes.
- Stir in the diced tomatoes (with their juice), kidney beans, small pasta, vegetable broth, dried basil, and dried oregano.
- Season with salt and pepper to taste. Bring the soup to a boil.
- Reduce the heat to low, cover the pot, and simmer for about 15-20 minutes, or

until the pasta is cooked and the vegetables are tender.

+ Taste and adjust the seasonings if necessary.

+ Serve the Minestrone soup hot, garnished with grated Parmesan cheese and fresh basil leaves if desired.

Spinach and Strawberry Salad

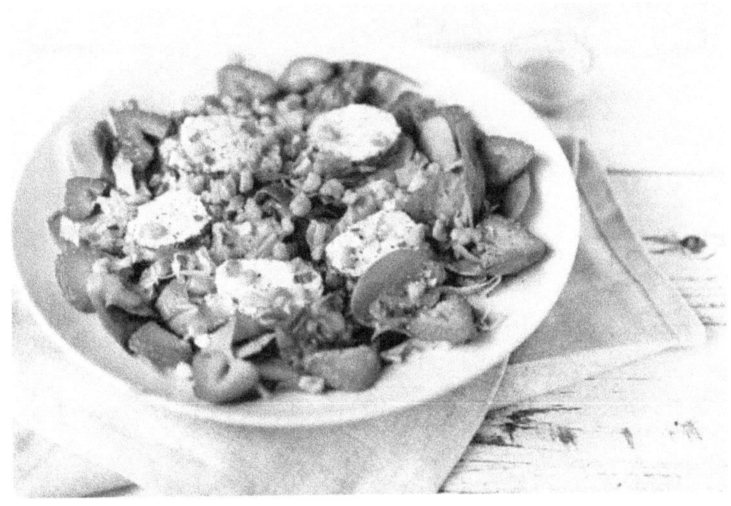

Ingredients:

+ 6 cups fresh baby spinach leaves

+ 1 1/2 cups fresh strawberries, sliced

+ 1/4 cup red onion, thinly sliced

+ 1/4 cup sliced almonds, toasted

+ 1/4 cup crumbled feta cheese (optional)

+ Balsamic vinaigrette dressing (store-bought or homemade)

Instructions:

+ In a large salad bowl, combine the fresh baby spinach leaves, sliced strawberries, and thinly sliced red onion.

+ Sprinkle the toasted sliced almonds over the salad.

+ If desired, add crumbled feta cheese for extra flavor.

+ Just before serving, drizzle balsamic vinaigrette dressing over the salad and toss gently to coat the ingredients evenly.

+ Serve your spinach and strawberry salad as a refreshing and healthy side dish or a light meal.

Lentil and Vegetable Stew

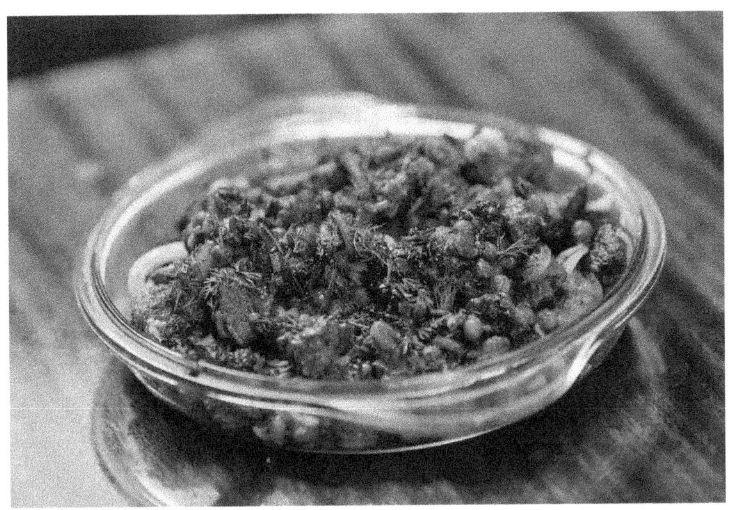

Ingredients:

- 1 cup dried green or brown lentils, rinsed and drained
- 4 cups vegetable broth (low-sodium)
- 1 onion, chopped
- 2 carrots, chopped
- 2 celery stalks, chopped
- 2 cloves garlic, minced

- 1 (14.5-ounce) can diced tomatoes
- 1 teaspoon dried thyme
- 1 teaspoon dried rosemary
- Salt and pepper to taste
- Fresh parsley, chopped (optional for garnish).

Instructions:

- In a large soup pot, combine the dried lentils and vegetable broth. Bring to a boil.
- Reduce the heat to low, cover, and simmer for about 15 minutes.
- Add the chopped onion, carrots, celery, and minced garlic to the pot. Continue to simmer for another 15-20 minutes,

or until the lentils and vegetables are tender.

- Stir in the diced tomatoes (with their juice), dried thyme, dried rosemary, salt, and pepper.
- Simmer for an additional 10 minutes to allow the flavors to meld.
- Taste and adjust the seasonings if needed.
- Serve the lentil and vegetable stew hot, garnished with chopped fresh parsley if desired.

Caesar Salad with Grilled Chicken

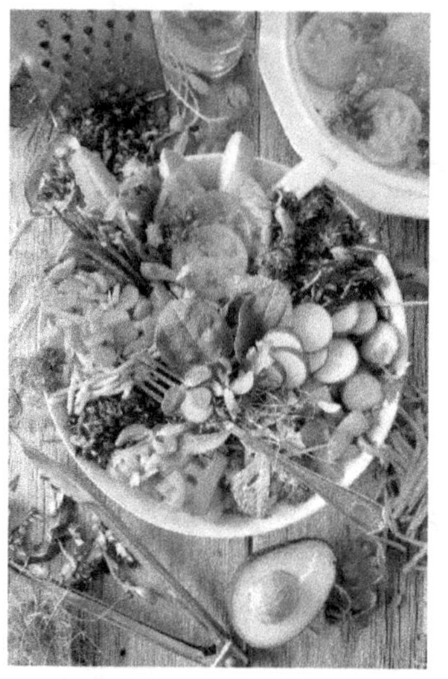

Ingredients:

- 2 boneless, skinless chicken breasts
- 1 tablespoon olive oil
- Salt and black pepper to taste
- 1 head of romaine lettuce, chopped
- 1/4 cup grated Parmesan cheese
- 1/4 cup croutons (look for whole grain options)
- Caesar salad dressing (store-bought or homemade)

Instructions:

- Preheat a grill or grill pan to medium-high heat.

- Rub the chicken breasts with olive oil and season with salt and black pepper.

- Grill the chicken for approximately 6-8 minutes per side, or until the internal temperature reaches 165°F (74°C) and the chicken is cooked through.

- Remove the grilled chicken from the grill and let it rest for a few minutes before slicing it into strips.

- In a large salad bowl, combine the chopped romaine lettuce, grated Parmesan cheese, and croutons.

- Add the grilled chicken strips on top of the salad.

- Drizzle Caesar salad dressing over the salad, and toss gently to coat the ingredients.
- Serve your Caesar salad with grilled chicken as a satisfying and protein-rich meal.

Butternut Squash Soup

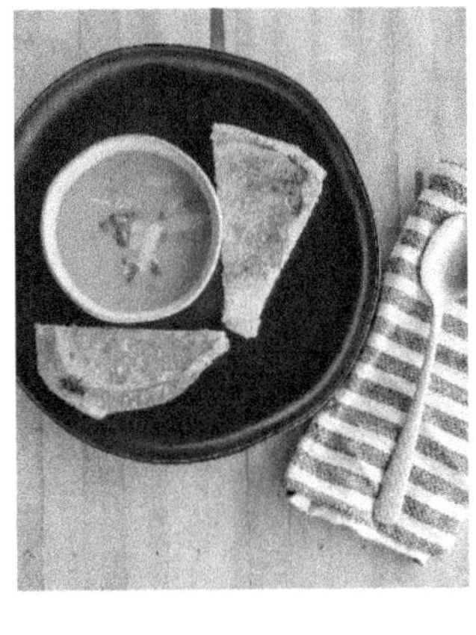

Ingredients:

- 1 medium butternut squash, peeled, seeded, and cubed
- 1 onion, chopped
- 2 carrots, chopped
- 2 celery stalks, chopped
- 2 cloves garlic, minced
- 4 cups vegetable broth (low-sodium)
- 1/2 teaspoon ground cinnamon
- 1/4 teaspoon ground nutmeg
- Salt and black pepper to taste
- 2 tablespoons olive oil
- Fresh thyme leaves (optional for garnish)

Instructions:

+ In a large pot, heat the olive oil over medium heat.

+ Add the chopped onion, carrots, celery, and minced garlic. Sauté for about 5-7 minutes until the vegetables begin to soften.

+ Add the cubed butternut squash, ground cinnamon, and ground nutmeg to the pot. Sauté for an additional 2-3 minutes to infuse the spices.

+ Pour in the vegetable broth and bring the mixture to a boil.

+ Reduce the heat to low, cover the pot, and simmer for approximately 20-25 minutes, or until the butternut squash and vegetables are tender.

+ Use an immersion blender or a regular blender to puree the soup until smooth and creamy. Be cautious when blending hot liquids.

+ Season the soup with salt and black pepper to taste.

+ Reheat the soup if needed, and serve hot, garnished with fresh thyme leaves if desired.

Main Courses

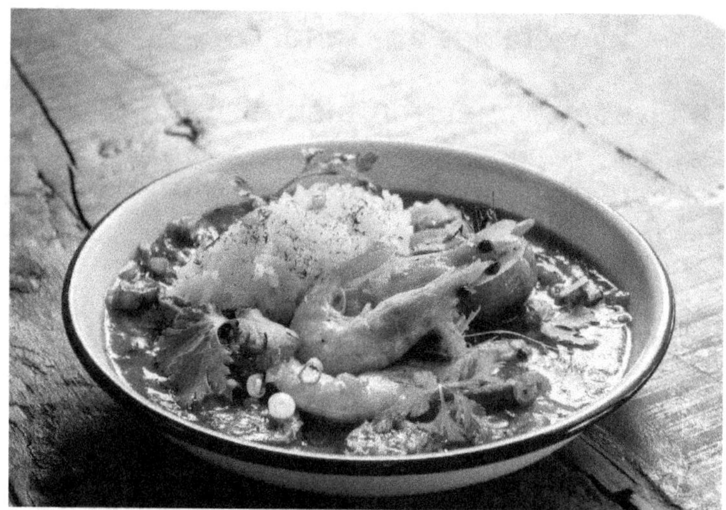

The most substantial or most significant dish during a meal where various courses are presented separately:

Grilled Salmon with Lemon-Dill Sauce

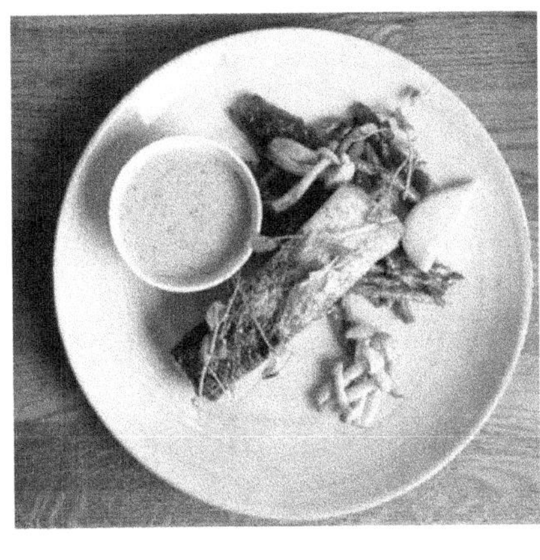

Ingredients:

- 4 salmon fillets
- 2 tablespoons olive oil
- Salt and black pepper to taste
- 2 tablespoons fresh lemon juice
- 2 tablespoons fresh dill, chopped
- Lemon wedges for garnish

Instructions:

- Preheat your grill to medium-high heat.
- Brush the salmon fillets with olive oil and season with salt and black pepper.

- Place the salmon fillets on the grill and cook for about 4-5 minutes per side, or until the salmon is opaque and flakes easily with a fork.

- While the salmon is grilling, prepare the lemon-dill sauce. In a small bowl, combine the fresh lemon juice and chopped fresh dill.

- Remove the grilled salmon from the heat and drizzle the lemon-dill sauce over the top.

- Garnish with lemon wedges and extra dill if desired.

- Serve your grilled salmon with lemon-dill sauce hot, accompanied by your choice of side dishes.

Chicken and Broccoli Stir-Fry

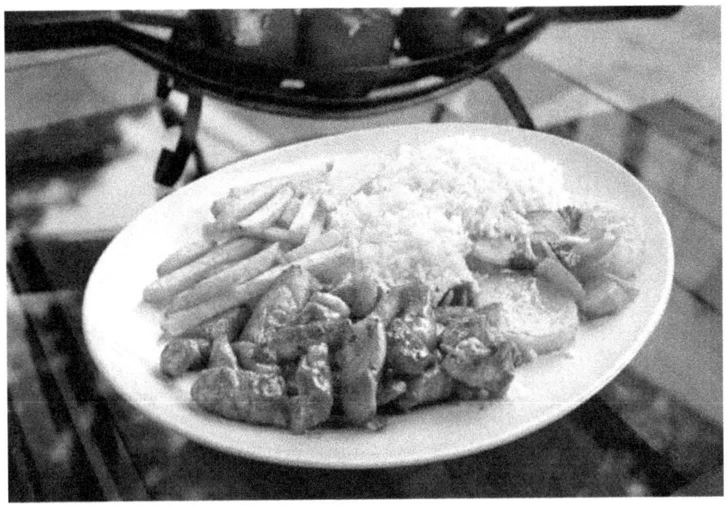

Ingredients:

+ 2 boneless, skinless chicken breasts, cut into bite-sized pieces

+ 2 cups broccoli florets

+ 1 red bell pepper, thinly sliced

+ 1/4 cup low-sodium soy sauce

+ 2 tablespoons honey or a sugar substitute

+ 2 cloves garlic, minced

+ 1 teaspoon fresh ginger, minced

+ 1 tablespoon cornstarch

+ 2 tablespoons vegetable oil

+ Cooked quinoa or brown rice (for serving)

Instructions:

+ In a small bowl, whisk together the low-sodium soy sauce, honey (or sugar substitute), minced garlic, minced ginger, and cornstarch. Set the sauce aside.

+ Heat the vegetable oil in a large skillet or wok over medium-high heat.

- Add the chicken pieces and stir-fry for 4-5 minutes, or until they are cooked through and no longer pink. Remove the chicken from the skillet and set it aside.

- In the same skillet, add the broccoli florets and sliced red bell pepper. Stir-fry for about 3-4 minutes, or until the vegetables are tender-crisp.

- Return the cooked chicken to the skillet and pour the sauce over the chicken and vegetables.

- Stir-fry for an additional 2-3 minutes, or until the sauce thickens and coats the ingredients evenly.

- Serve the chicken and broccoli stir-fry over cooked quinoa or brown rice.

Quinoa and Black Bean Bowl

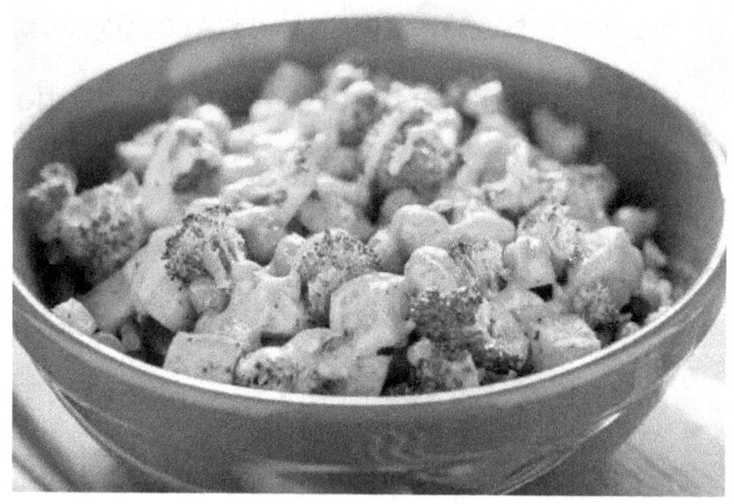

Ingredients:

- 1 cup quinoa, rinsed and drained
- 2 cups vegetable broth (low-sodium)
- 1 (15-ounce) can black beans, drained and rinsed
- 1 cup corn kernels (fresh, frozen, or canned)
- 1 red bell pepper, diced

- 1/2 red onion, finely chopped
- 1/4 cup fresh cilantro, chopped
- 1 avocado, diced
- Lime wedges for garnish

Instructions:

- In a saucepan, combine the quinoa and vegetable broth. Bring to a boil, then reduce the heat to low, cover, and simmer for about 15 minutes, or until the quinoa is cooked and the liquid is absorbed.
- Fluff the cooked quinoa with a fork and let it cool slightly.
- In a large bowl, combine the cooked quinoa, black beans, corn kernels, diced

red bell pepper, and finely chopped red onion.

- Stir in the chopped fresh cilantro.
- Divide the quinoa and black bean mixture into serving bowls.
- Top each bowl with diced avocado and garnish with lime wedges.
- Serve your quinoa and black bean bowls as a wholesome and filling main course.

Spaghetti Squash with Marinara

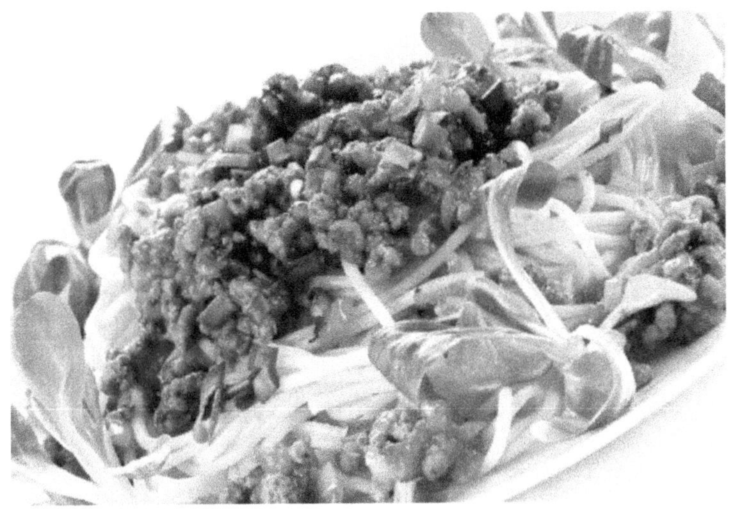

<u>Ingredients:</u>

+ 1 medium spaghetti squash

+ 2 cups marinara sauce (store-bought or homemade)

+ 1/4 cup grated Parmesan cheese (optional for garnish)

+ Fresh basil leaves (optional for garnish)

Instructions:

- Preheat your oven to 375°F (190°C).

- Carefully cut the spaghetti squash in half lengthwise and remove the seeds and pulp.

- Place the squash halves, cut side down, on a baking sheet lined with parchment paper.

- Bake in the preheated oven for about 30-40 minutes, or until the squash flesh is tender and easily shreds into "spaghetti" with a fork.

- While the squash is baking, heat the marinara sauce in a saucepan over medium heat until it's warmed through.

- Once the squash is done, remove it from the oven and use a fork to scrape the flesh into "spaghetti" strands.

- Serve the spaghetti squash with marinara sauce, and if desired, garnish with grated Parmesan cheese and fresh basil leaves.

- Enjoy this low-carb alternative to traditional pasta!

Tofu and Vegetable Curry

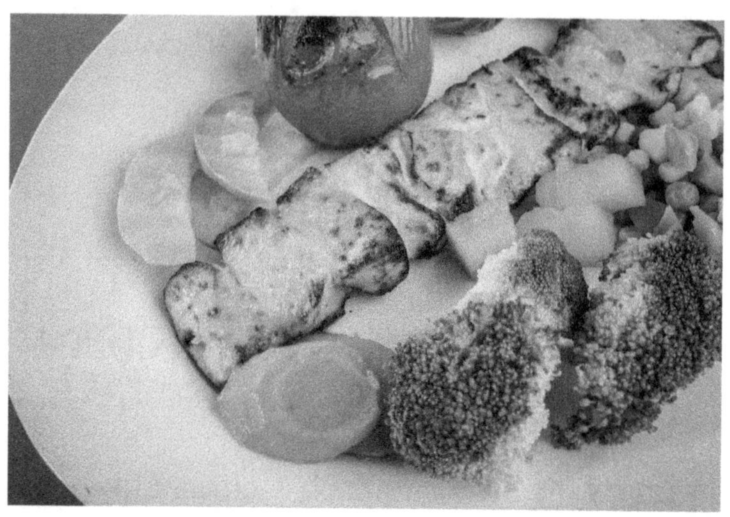

Ingredients:

- 1 block of extra-firm tofu, cubed
- 2 cups mixed vegetables (e.g., bell peppers, broccoli, carrots)
- 1 can (14 ounces) of coconut milk
- 2 tablespoons red curry paste
- 1 tablespoon soy sauce (low-sodium)
- 1 tablespoon vegetable oil

- I tablespoon brown sugar or a sugar substitute
- Fresh cilantro leaves for garnish
- Cooked brown rice (for serving)

Instructions:

- In a large skillet or wok, heat the vegetable oil over medium-high heat.
- Add the cubed tofu and cook until it's lightly browned on all sides. Remove the tofu from the skillet and set it aside.
- In the same skillet, add the mixed vegetables and stir-fry for about 3-4 minutes, or until they begin to soften.
- Stir in the red curry paste and cook for another minute to release its flavors.

- Add the cooked tofu back to the skillet and pour in the coconut milk, soy sauce, and brown sugar.
- Stir to combine all the ingredients and simmer for 5-7 minutes, or until the sauce thickens slightly.
- Taste and adjust the seasonings if necessary.
- Serve the tofu and vegetable curry hot over cooked brown rice, garnished with fresh cilantro leaves.

Sides and Accompaniments

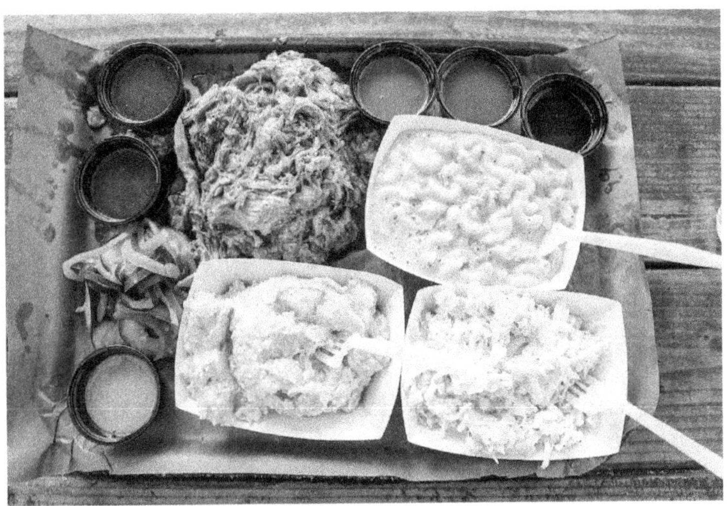

We serve side dishes as a complement to our main courses. Salads, stir-fries, gravies, curries, dips, fritters, pickles, and jams are just a few examples. It may be made from either meat or vegetables. In essence, they make it easier for us to eat our main courses.

Garlic Roasted Brussels Sprouts

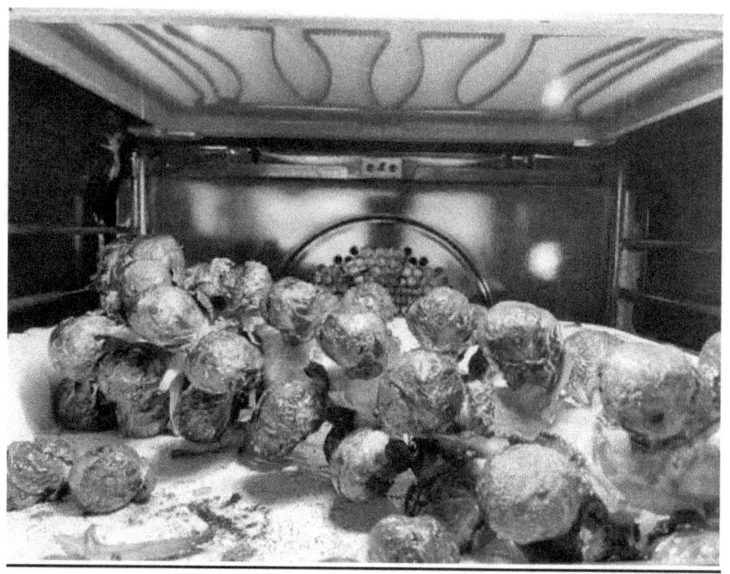

<u>Ingredients:</u>

+ 1-pound Brussels sprouts, trimmed and halved

+ 2 tablespoons olive oil

+ 3 cloves garlic, minced

+ Salt and black pepper to taste

+ Lemon zest (optional for garnish)

<u>Instructions:</u>

- Preheat your oven to 400°F (200°C).

- In a large bowl, toss the halved Brussels sprouts with olive oil, minced garlic, salt, and black pepper until they are evenly coated.

- Spread the Brussels sprouts in a single layer on a baking sheet lined with parchment paper.

- Roast in the preheated oven for about 25-30 minutes, or until the Brussels sprouts are tender and lightly browned, stirring once halfway through.

- Remove from the oven and garnish with lemon zest if desired.

+ Serve your garlic roasted Brussels sprouts hot as a flavorful side dish.

Brown Rice Pilaf

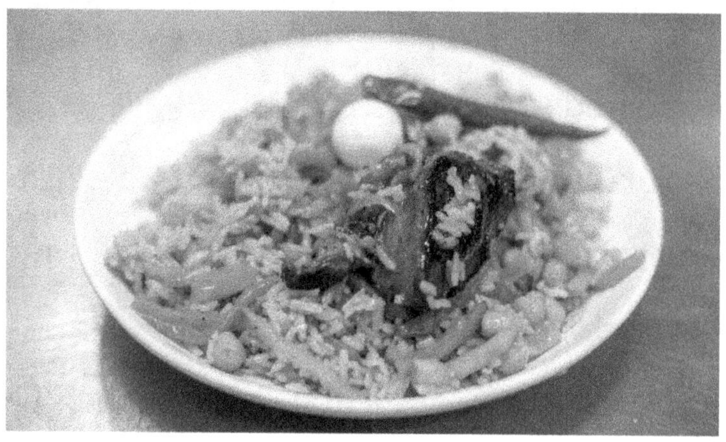

Ingredients:

+ 1 cup brown rice

+ 2 cups vegetable broth (low-sodium)

+ 1/4 cup finely chopped onion

+ 1/4 cup chopped bell pepper (red, green, or yellow)

- 1/4 cup chopped celery

- 1/4 cup chopped carrots

- 2 cloves garlic, minced

- 1 tablespoon olive oil

- 1/2 teaspoon dried thyme

- Salt and black pepper to taste

- Chopped fresh parsley for garnish (optional)

Instructions:

- In a large saucepan, heat the olive oil over medium heat.

- Add the finely chopped onion, chopped bell pepper, chopped celery, and chopped carrots. Sauté for about 5-7 minutes, or until the vegetables begin to soften.

+ Stir in the minced garlic and dried thyme, and cook for another minute to release their flavors.

+ Add the brown rice to the saucepan and cook for 1-2 minutes, stirring to coat the rice with the vegetables and oil.

+ Pour in the vegetable broth, season with salt and black pepper to taste, and bring to a boil.

+ Reduce the heat to low, cover the saucepan, and simmer for about 45-50 minutes, or until the rice is tender and the liquid is absorbed.

+ Fluff the cooked brown rice with a fork.

＋ Garnish with chopped fresh parsley if desired.

＋ Serve your brown rice pilaf as a wholesome and hearty side dish.

Mashed Cauliflower

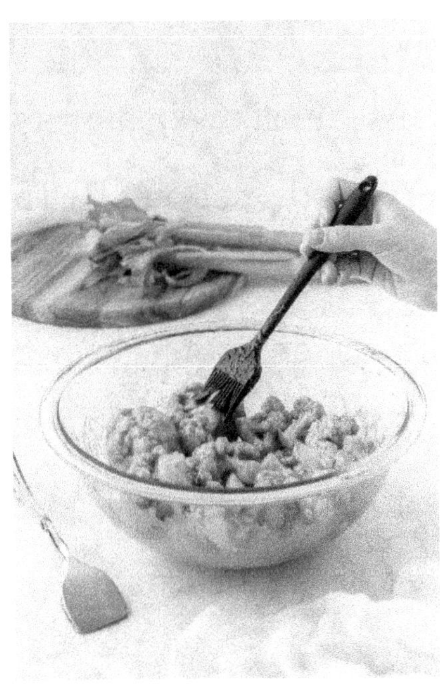

Ingredients:

＋ 1 head of cauliflower, cut into florets

＋ 2 cloves garlic, minced

＋ 2 tablespoons plain Greek yogurt

- 2 tablespoons grated Parmesan cheese (optional)
- Salt and black pepper to taste
- Chopped fresh chives for garnish (optional)

Instructions:

- Steam or boil the cauliflower florets until they are very tender, about 10-15 minutes.
- Drain the cauliflower and place it in a food processor.
- Add the minced garlic, plain Greek yogurt, and grated Parmesan cheese (if using).

- Season with salt and black pepper to taste.
- Process until the cauliflower is smooth and has the consistency of mashed potatoes.
- Taste and adjust the seasonings if needed.
- Transfer the mashed cauliflower to a serving dish.
- Garnish with chopped fresh chives if desired.
- Serve your mashed cauliflower as a low-carb alternative to traditional mashed potatoes.

Steamed Asparagus with Almonds

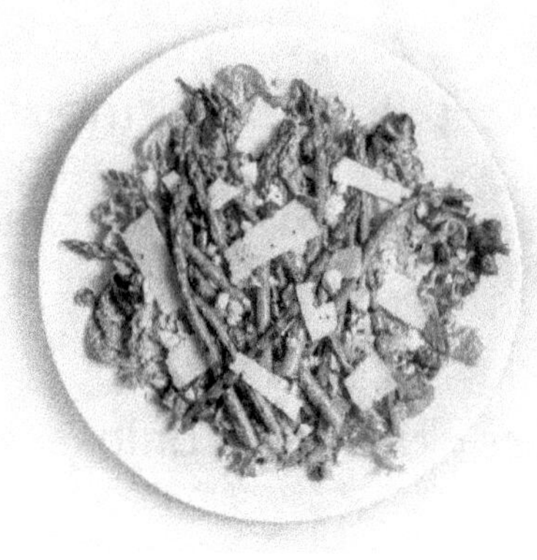

Ingredients:

- 1 bunch of fresh asparagus spears, trimmed
- 2 tablespoons slivered almonds, toasted
- 1 tablespoon olive oil
- 1 teaspoon lemon juice
- Salt and black pepper to taste
- Lemon zest (optional for garnish)

Instructions:

- Steam the trimmed asparagus spears until they are tender-crisp, about 4-5 minutes.
- In a small skillet, toast the slivered almonds over medium heat until they are lightly golden, stirring frequently.
- In a bowl, whisk together the olive oil and lemon juice.
- Season with salt and black pepper to taste.
- Drizzle the lemon-oil mixture over the steamed asparagus.
- Top with toasted slivered almonds and garnish with lemon zest if desired.

✦ Serve your steamed asparagus with almonds hot as a nutritious side dish.

Roasted Root Vegetables

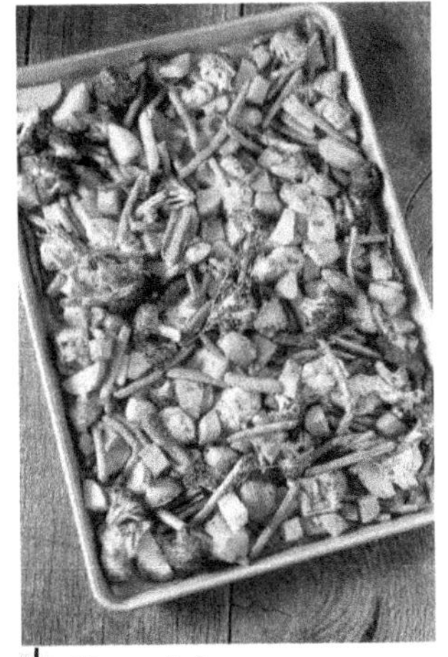

Ingredients:

- 3 cups mixed root vegetables (e.g., carrots, parsnips, sweet potatoes, beets), peeled and diced
- 2 tablespoons olive oil
- 1 teaspoon dried thyme
- 1 teaspoon dried rosemary
- Salt and black pepper to taste
- Fresh parsley leaves for garnish (optional)

Instructions:

- Preheat your oven to 425°F (220°C).

- In a large bowl, toss the diced root vegetables with olive oil, dried thyme, dried rosemary, salt, and black pepper until they are evenly coated.

- Spread the seasoned root vegetables in a single layer on a baking sheet lined with parchment paper.

- Roast in the preheated oven for about 25-30 minutes, or until the vegetables are tender and caramelized, stirring once halfway through.

- Remove from the oven and garnish with fresh parsley leaves if desired.

- Serve your roasted root vegetables as a flavorful and colorful side dish.

Desert

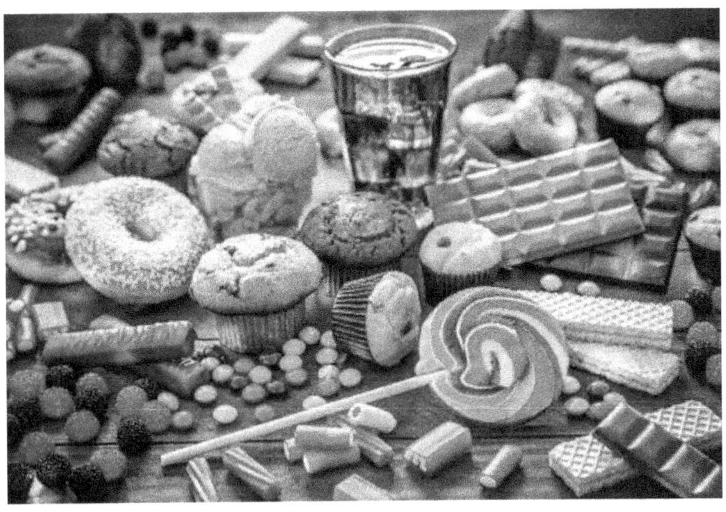

Since fruit is naturally sweet, the term "dessert" can be used to describe a wide range of sweets, including fruit salad, biscuits, cakes, cookies, custards, gelatins, ice creams, pastries, pies, puddings, macaroons, and sweet soups.

Berry and Greek Yogurt Parfait

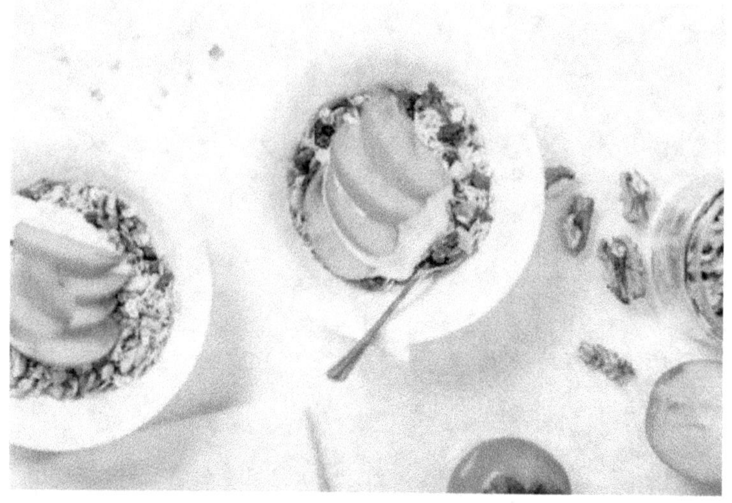

Ingredients:

- 1 cup fresh mixed berries (e.g., strawberries, blueberries, raspberries)
- 1 cup plain Greek yogurt
- 2 tablespoons honey or a sugar substitute
- 1/4 cup granola (look for a low-sugar option)

✦ Fresh mint leaves for garnish (optional)

Instructions:

✦ In a serving glass or bowl, layer half of the plain Greek yogurt at the bottom.

✦ Add half of the fresh mixed berries on top of the yogurt.

✦ Drizzle with 1 tablespoon of honey (or sugar substitute) for sweetness.

✦ Repeat the layers with the remaining yogurt, berries, and honey.

✦ Sprinkle granola on the top layer for a crunchy texture.

✦ Garnish with fresh mint leaves if desired.

- Serve your berry and Greek yogurt parfait chilled as a delicious and healthy dessert.

Baked Apple with Cinnamon

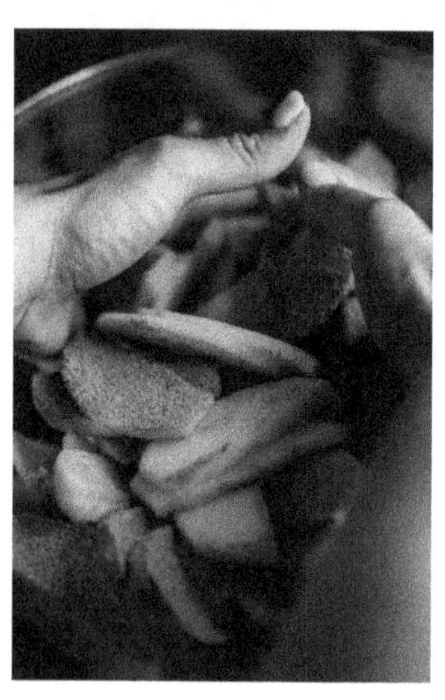

Ingredients:

- 2 apples (e.g., Granny Smith or Honeycrisp)
- 1 teaspoon ground cinnamon
- 1/4 teaspoon ground nutmeg
- 2 teaspoons honey or a sugar substitute
- Chopped nuts (e.g., walnuts or almonds) for garnish (optional)

+ Greek yogurt (optional for serving)

Instructions:

+ Preheat your oven to 375°F (190°C).

+ Wash and core the apples, removing the seeds and creating a small well in the center.

+ In a small bowl, mix together the ground cinnamon and ground nutmeg.

+ Sprinkle the cinnamon-nutmeg mixture evenly over the apples.

+ Drizzle 1 teaspoon of honey (or sugar substitute) over each apple.

+ Place the apples in a baking dish and add a small amount of water to the bottom of the dish to prevent sticking.

- Bake in the preheated oven for 25-30 minutes, or until the apples are tender and can be easily pierced with a fork.
- Remove from the oven and let cool slightly.
- If desired, garnish with chopped nuts and serve with a dollop of Greek yogurt.

Dark Chocolate-Dipped Strawberries

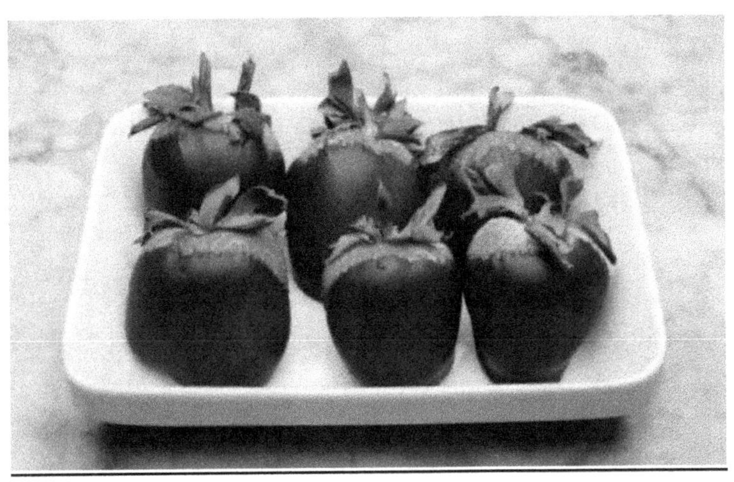

Ingredients:

- 1 cup fresh strawberries, washed and dried
- 2 ounces dark chocolate (70% cocoa or higher)
- 1 teaspoon coconut oil (optional for smoother chocolate)

<u>**Instructions:**</u>

- Line a baking sheet with parchment paper.

- In a microwave-safe bowl, melt the dark chocolate in 20-second intervals, stirring between each interval until the chocolate is smooth. If desired, add coconut oil to the chocolate for a smoother consistency.

- Hold each strawberry by the stem and dip it into the melted dark chocolate, coating it about halfway.

- Place the chocolate-dipped strawberries on the prepared baking sheet.

- Allow the chocolate to set by placing the baking sheet in the refrigerator for about 15-20 minutes.
- Once the chocolate is firm, transfer the dark chocolate-dipped strawberries to a serving plate.
- Serve as a delightful and guilt-free dessert.

Chia Seed Pudding

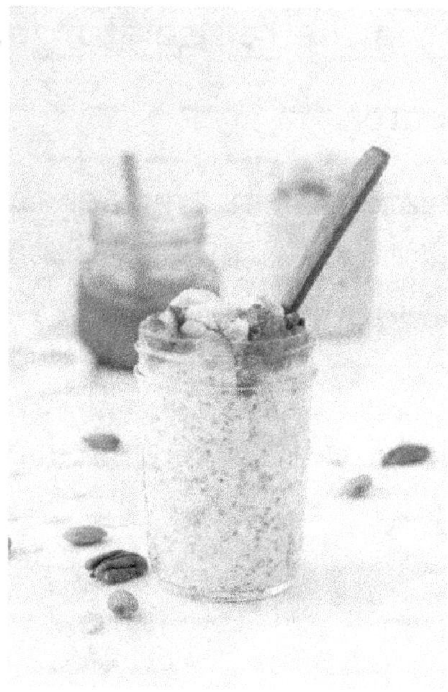

Ingredients:

- 1/4 cup chia seeds
- 1 cup unsweetened almond milk (or any milk of your choice)
- 1 tablespoon honey or a sugar substitute
- 1/2 teaspoon vanilla extract
- Fresh berries for topping (optional)

Instructions:

- In a bowl, combine the chia seeds, unsweetened almond milk, honey (or sugar substitute), and vanilla extract.
- Stir well to mix all the ingredients.
- Cover the bowl and refrigerate for at least 4 hours or overnight, allowing the chia seeds to absorb the liquid and thicken the pudding.
- Before serving, give the pudding a good stir.
- Top with fresh berries if desired.
- Enjoy your chia seed pudding as a nutritious and satisfying dessert.

Sugar-Free Pumpkin Pie

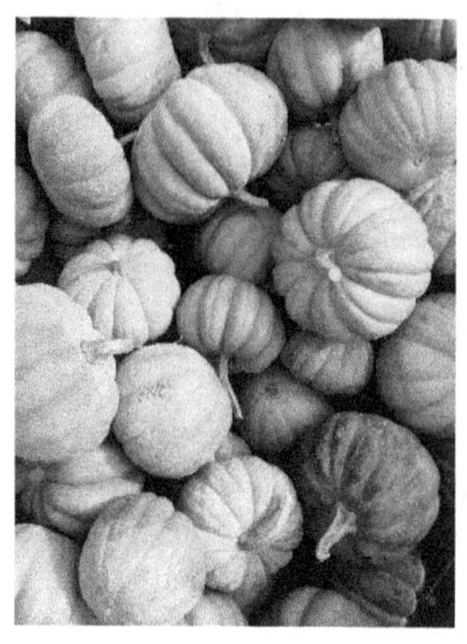

Ingredients:

+ 1 pre-made sugar-free graham cracker pie crust
+ 1 can (15 ounces) pumpkin puree (not pumpkin pie filling)
+ 1 cup unsweetened almond milk (or any milk of your choice)
+ 2 large eggs
+ 1 teaspoon ground cinnamon
+ 1/2 teaspoon ground nutmeg
+ 1/4 teaspoon ground cloves
+ 1/4 teaspoon ground ginger

- 1/4 cup sugar substitute (e.g., Stevia or erythritol)
- Whipped cream (sugar-free) for topping (optional)

Instructions:

- Preheat your oven to 375°F (190°C).
- In a large bowl, whisk together the pumpkin puree, unsweetened almond milk, large eggs, ground cinnamon, ground nutmeg, ground cloves, ground ginger, and sugar substitute until well combined.
- Pour the pumpkin mixture into the sugar-free graham cracker pie crust.

- Bake in the preheated oven for 45-50 minutes, or until the filling is set and a toothpick inserted into the center comes out clean.
- Remove the pumpkin pie from the oven and let it cool completely.
- If desired, top with sugar-free whipped cream before serving.
- Slice and enjoy your sugar-free pumpkin pie as a delicious dessert with the flavors of fall.

Beverages

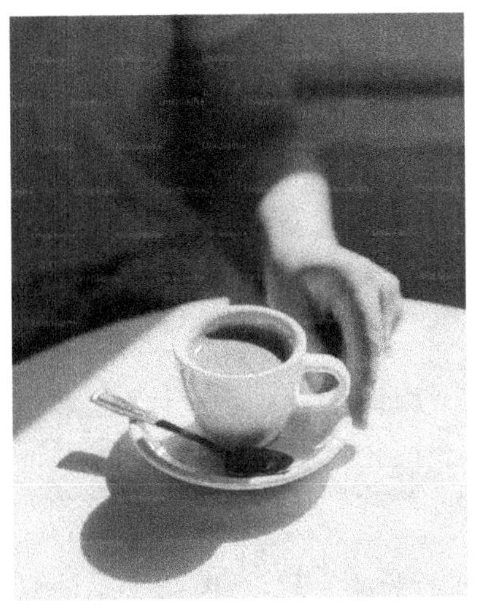

A liquid meant for human consumption is referred to as a drink or beverage. Drinks serve the simple purpose of quenching thirst, but they also have significant cultural meanings. Plain water, milk, juice, smoothies, and soft drinks are examples of common drinks.

Green Smoothie

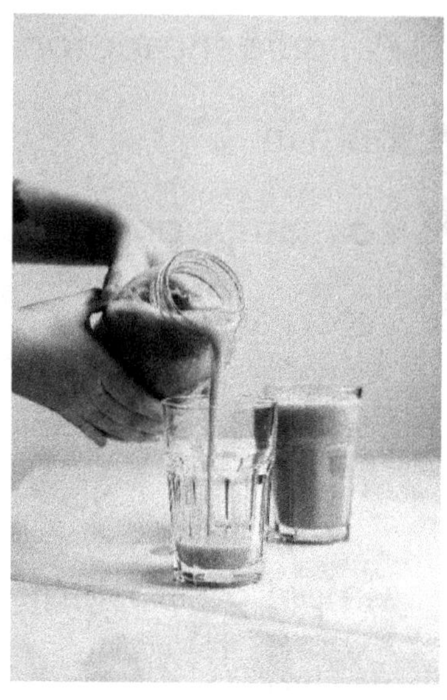

Ingredients:

+ 1 cup fresh spinach leaves
+ 1/2 cup chopped cucumber
+ 1/2 banana
+ 1/2 cup unsweetened almond milk (or any milk of your choice)
+ 1/2 cup plain Greek yogurt
+ 1 tablespoon honey or a sugar substitute (optional)
+ Ice cubes (optional)
+ Fresh mint leaves for garnish (optional)

Instructions:

- Place the fresh spinach leaves, chopped cucumber, banana, unsweetened almond milk, and plain Greek yogurt in a blender.
- If you prefer a sweeter smoothie, add honey (or sugar substitute) to taste.
- Optionally, add ice cubes for a colder and thicker texture.
- Blend until the ingredients are smooth and well combined.
- Taste and adjust sweetness or consistency if needed.
- Pour the green smoothie into a glass.
- Garnish with fresh mint leaves if desired.

+ Serve your green smoothie as a nutritious and refreshing beverage.

Infused Water with Citrus

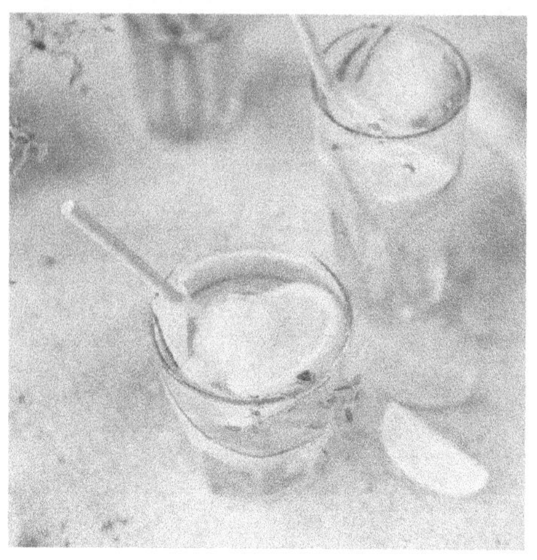

Ingredients:

+ 1 lemon, thinly sliced
+ 1 lime, thinly sliced
+ 1 orange, thinly sliced
+ 1/2 cucumber, thinly sliced
+ Fresh mint leaves
+ Ice cubes
+ Water

Instructions:

- In a large pitcher, combine the thinly sliced lemon, lime, orange, and cucumber.
- Add a handful of fresh mint leaves to the pitcher.
- Fill the pitcher with ice cubes.
- Pour water over the ice and sliced fruits.
- Stir gently to combine the ingredients.
- Refrigerate for at least 1 hour to allow the flavors to infuse.
- Serve the infused water with citrus in glasses, garnished with extra mint leaves and ice cubes if desired.
- Enjoy this refreshing and hydrating beverage.

Iced Herbal Tea

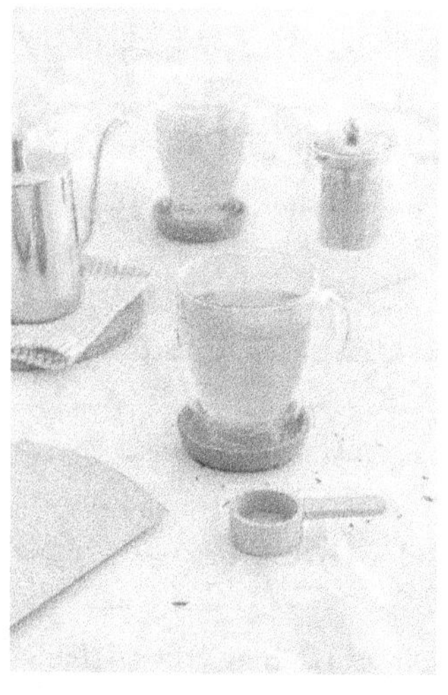

Ingredients:

- 2 herbal tea bags (e.g., chamomile, peppermint, hibiscus)
- 2 cups boiling water
- 1-2 teaspoons honey or a sugar substitute (optional)
- Slices of lemon or lime (optional)
- Fresh herbs (e.g., mint or basil) for garnish (optional)
- Ice cubes

Instructions:

- Place the herbal tea bags in a heatproof pitcher or container.
- Pour boiling water over the tea bags.
- Let the tea steep for the recommended time (usually 5-7 minutes, but follow the instructions on the tea package).
- If desired, add honey (or sugar substitute) to sweeten the tea while it's still hot and stir to dissolve.
- Remove the tea bags and let the tea cool to room temperature.
- Refrigerate the tea until it's chilled.
- To serve, fill glasses with ice cubes and pour the chilled herbal tea over the ice.

+ Garnish with slices of lemon or lime and fresh herbs if desired.

+ Enjoy your iced herbal tea as a calming and refreshing beverage.

Berry Blast Protein Shake

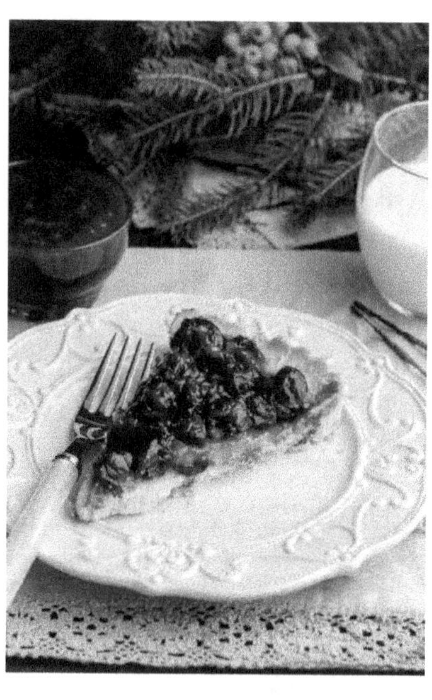

Ingredients:

+ 1 cup unsweetened almond milk (or any milk of your choice)

+ 1/2 cup plain Greek yogurt

- 1/2 cup mixed berries (e.g., strawberries, blueberries, raspberries)
- 1 scoop of your favorite protein powder (low-sugar)
- 1 tablespoon chia seeds (optional for added fiber)
- 1/2 teaspoon vanilla extract
- Ice cubes (optional)
- Fresh berries for garnish (optional)
- Instructions:

- In a blender, combine the unsweetened almond milk, plain Greek yogurt, mixed berries, protein powder, chia seeds (if using), and vanilla extract.

- Optionally, add ice cubes for a colder and thicker shake.
- Blend until the ingredients are smooth and well combined.
- Taste and adjust sweetness or consistency if needed.
- Pour the berry blast protein shake into a glass.
- Garnish with fresh berries if desired.
- Serve your protein-packed shake as a satisfying and energizing beverage.

Cucumber-Mint Cooler

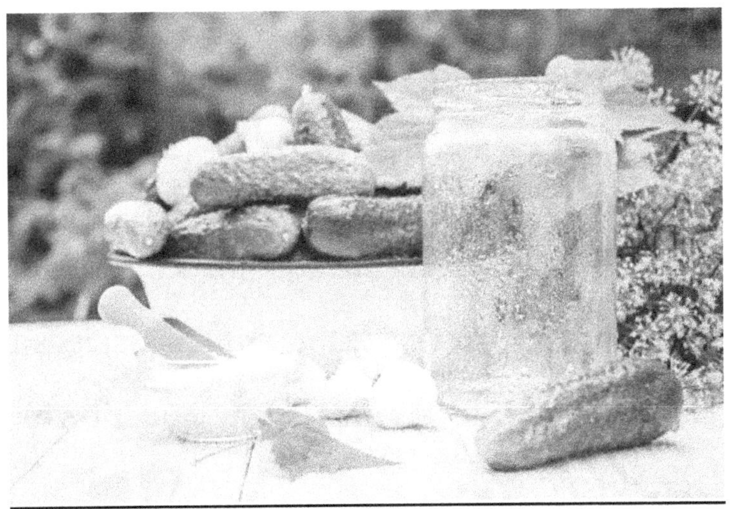

Ingredients:

- 1 cucumber, peeled and sliced
- 1/4 cup fresh mint leaves
- 2 tablespoons fresh lime juice
- 1 tablespoon honey or a sugar substitute
- 2 cups cold water
- Ice cubes

+ Lime wedges and mint sprigs for garnish (optional)

Instructions:

+ In a blender, combine the peeled and sliced cucumber, fresh mint leaves, fresh lime juice, honey (or sugar substitute), and cold water.
+ Blend until the mixture is smooth and the flavors are well combined.
+ Taste and adjust sweetness or lime juice if needed.
+ Fill glasses with ice cubes.
+ Pour the cucumber-mint cooler over the ice.

+ Optionally, garnish with lime wedges and mint sprigs.

+ Serve your cucumber-mint cooler as a refreshing and revitalizing beverage.

SPECIAL OCCASION RECIPES

Grilled Vegetable Platter

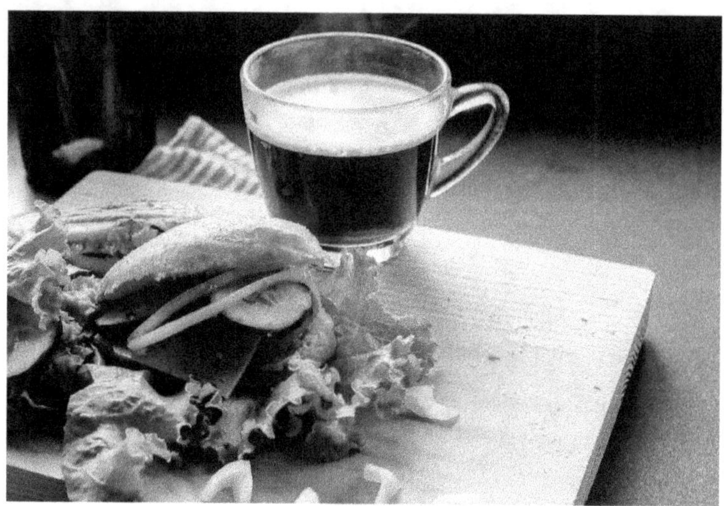

Ingredients:

+ Assorted vegetables (e.g., bell peppers, zucchini, eggplant, mushrooms, cherry tomatoes)

+ Olive oil

+ Salt and black pepper to taste

- Fresh herbs (e.g., thyme, rosemary, basil) for garnish (optional)
- Balsamic vinegar (optional for drizzling)

Instructions:

- Preheat your grill to medium-high heat.
- Wash and prepare the assorted vegetables by slicing them into appropriate sizes for grilling.
- Brush the vegetables with olive oil and season with salt and black pepper.
- Place the vegetables on the grill and cook, turning occasionally, until they are tender and have grill marks (usually 5-10 minutes, depending on the vegetable).

+ Remove the grilled vegetables from the heat and arrange them on a platter.

+ Optionally, drizzle with balsamic vinegar and garnish with fresh herbs.

+ Serve your grilled vegetable platter as a colorful and flavorful side dish for special occasions.

Herb-Roasted Turkey

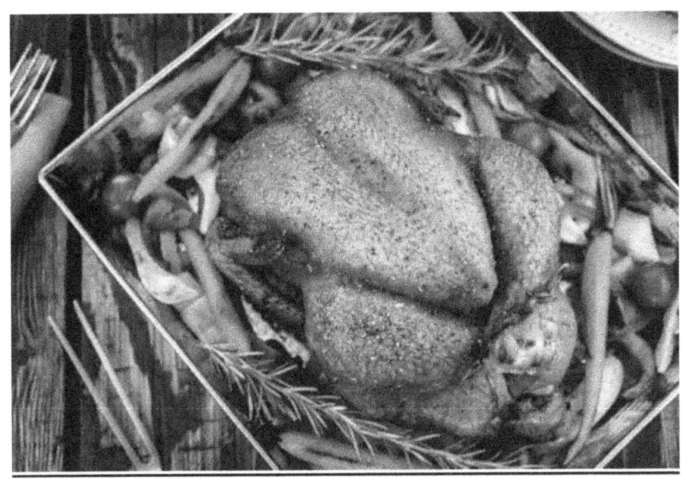

Ingredients:

- 1 whole turkey (size according to your needs)
- Olive oil
- Fresh herbs (e.g., rosemary, thyme, sage)
- Salt and black pepper to taste
- Garlic cloves (optional for extra flavor)

✦ Lemon wedges (optional for garnish)

Instructions:

✦ Preheat your oven to the appropriate temperature based on the size of your turkey (usually 325°F to 350°F or 160°C to 175°C).

✦ Rinse the turkey under cold water and pat it dry with paper towels.

✦ Rub the turkey with olive oil, and season generously with salt and black pepper, both inside and outside the cavity.

✦ Stuff the cavity of the turkey with fresh herbs and, if desired, garlic cloves and lemon wedges for added flavor.

- Place the turkey in a roasting pan, breast side up.
- Roast the turkey in the preheated oven, following the recommended cooking time based on the turkey's size (usually 13-15 minutes per pound).
- Baste the turkey with pan juices every 30 minutes to keep it moist.
- Use a meat thermometer to ensure the turkey reaches an internal temperature of 165°F (74°C) in the thickest part of the thigh.
- Once the turkey is done, remove it from the oven and let it rest for about 15-20 minutes before carving.

+ Carve and serve your herb-roasted turkey as the centerpiece of your special occasion meal.

Quinoa-Stuffed Bell Peppers

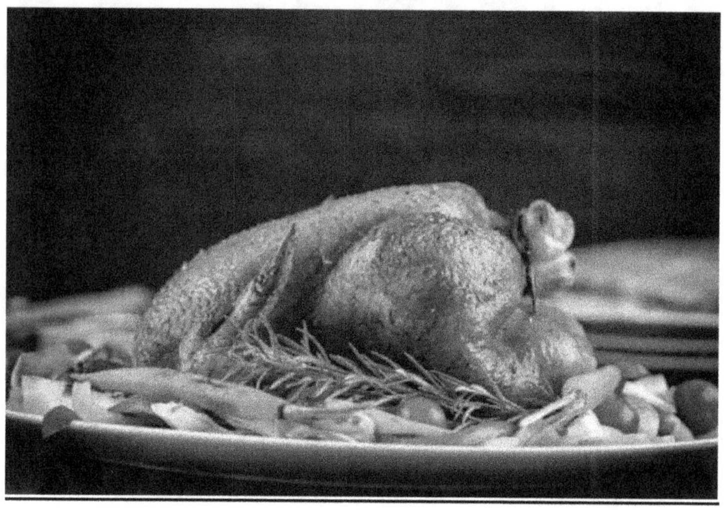

<u>Ingredients:</u>

+ 4 bell peppers (any color)

+ 1 cup quinoa, rinsed and drained

+ 2 cups vegetable broth (low-sodium)

- 1 can (15 ounces) black beans, drained and rinsed
- 1 cup corn kernels (fresh, frozen, or canned)
- 1 cup diced tomatoes (canned or fresh)
- 1/2 cup diced onion
- 2 cloves garlic, minced
- 1 teaspoon ground cumin
- Salt and black pepper to taste
- Shredded cheese (low-fat) for topping (optional)

Instructions:

- Preheat your oven to 375°F (190°C).
- Cut the tops off the bell peppers and remove the seeds and membranes.

- In a saucepan, combine the quinoa and vegetable broth. Bring to a boil, then reduce the heat to low, cover, and simmer for about 15 minutes, or until the quinoa is cooked and the liquid is absorbed.

- In a large bowl, combine the cooked quinoa, black beans, corn kernels, diced tomatoes, diced onion, minced garlic, ground cumin, salt, and black pepper. Mix well.

- Stuff each bell pepper with the quinoa mixture, pressing it down gently.

- Place the stuffed bell peppers in a baking dish.

+ Optionally, top each stuffed pepper with shredded cheese.

+ Cover the baking dish with foil and bake in the preheated oven for about 25-30 minutes, or until the peppers are tender.

+ Remove the foil and bake for an additional 5-10 minutes, or until the cheese (if used) is melted and bubbly.

+ Serve your quinoa-stuffed bell peppers as a wholesome and eye-catching main course for special occasions.

Cauliflower Mash with Gravy

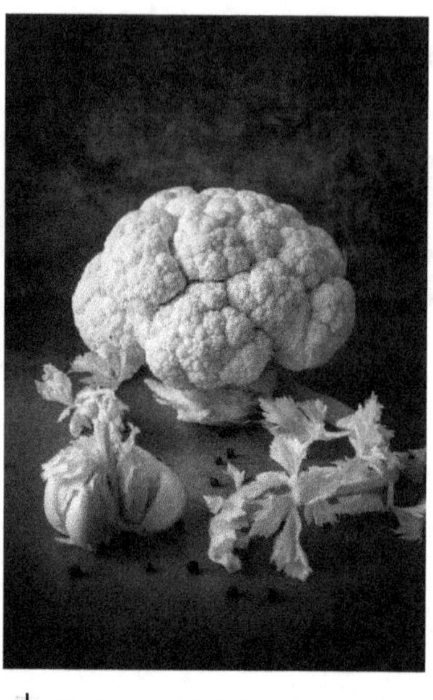

<u>Ingredients:</u>

+ 1 head of cauliflower, cut into florets
+ 2 cloves garlic, minced
+ 2 tablespoons plain Greek yogurt
+ Salt and black pepper to taste
+ Gravy (choose a low-sugar or sugar-free option)
+ Fresh parsley leaves for garnish (optional)

Instructions:

- Steam or boil the cauliflower florets until they are very tender, about 10-15 minutes.
- Drain the cauliflower and place it in a food processor.
- Add the minced garlic, plain Greek yogurt, salt, and black pepper.
- Process until the cauliflower is smooth and has the consistency of mashed potatoes.
- Taste and adjust the seasonings if needed.
- Warm the gravy in a saucepan over low heat.

- Serve the cauliflower mash with a drizzle of warm gravy.
- Optionally, garnish with fresh parsley leaves.
- Enjoy your cauliflower mash with gravy as a satisfying side dish for special occasions.

Fresh Fruit Salad

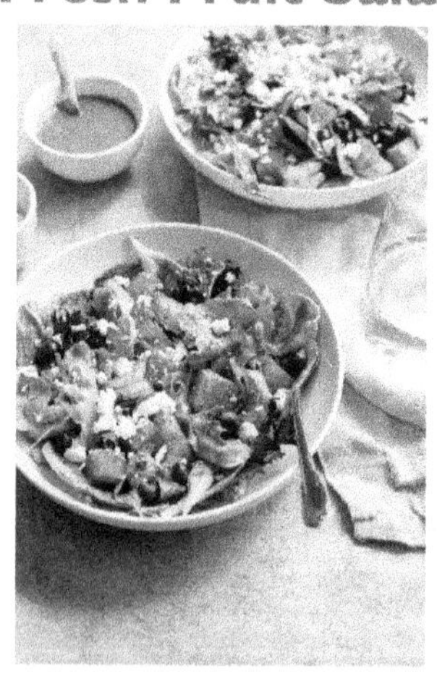

Ingredients:

- Assorted fresh fruits (e.g., berries, melons, citrus, grapes, pineapple)
- Fresh mint leaves for garnish (optional)

+ Honey or a sugar substitute for drizzling (optional)

Instructions:

+ Wash, peel (if necessary), and cut the assorted fresh fruits into bite-sized pieces.
+ Combine the fruits in a large serving bowl.
+ Optionally, drizzle honey (or sugar substitute) over the fruit salad for extra sweetness.
+ Gently toss the fruits to combine.
+ Garnish with fresh mint leaves if desired.

✦ Serve your fresh fruit salad as a naturally sweet and colorful dessert for special occasions.

Week after week Dinner Arranging Guide

Introduction:

- The significance of feast anticipating overseeing type 2 diabetes.
- Advantages of a week by week dinner plan, including better glucose control and better dietary patterns.

Steps for weekly Meal Planning:

Laying out objectives: Lay out unambiguous dietary objectives and focuses for the week.

Making a menu: Plan adjusted and nutritious feasts.

Composing a shopping list: Order a rundown of fixings required.

Getting ready feasts ahead of time: Save time by cooking bigger groups.

Putting away food securely: Tips on food capacity to keep up with newness.

Checking and changing: Monitor glucose levels and make vital changes.

Example Meal Planning:

An example week by week feast intend to assist perusers with getting everything rolling.

Segment Control Tips

Significance of Piece Control:

+ Understanding the effect of piece sizes on glucose and in general wellbeing.

+ Advantages of part control for weight the executives.

Segment Control Plans:

+ Use estimating cups and scales.

+ Obvious prompts: Contrasting bits with regular items.

+ Peruse food names.

+ Be careful while eating.

+ Share dishes at eateries.

+ More modest plates and utensils.

Rules for Healthy Ingredient Setting:

- Step by step instructions to settle on better fixing decisions while keeping up with flavor.

- Diminishing sugar, salt, and unfortunate fats.

Normal Ingredients Replacements:

- Sugar substitutes.

- Entire grains for refined grains.

- Greek yogurt for sharp cream or mayonnaise.

- Olive oil for spread or margarine.

- Spices and flavors for salt.

- Lean protein sources.

Feasting Out with Diabetes

Ways to eat Out:

- Prepare.

- Survey the menu on the web.

- Make unique solicitations.

- Share dishes.

- Be careful of sauces and dressings.

- Pick barbecued or simmered choices.

- Watch segment sizes.

- Limit liquor and treat.

Overseeing Glucose Levels

Blood Sugar Checking:

- The significance of ordinary glucose testing.

+ Instructions to decipher glucose readings.

+ When to contact a medical care supplier.

Way of life Elements:

+ The job of active work and stress the executives.

+ The meaning of rest and drug the executives.

Summary:

Key focus points and a sign of the significance of proactive administration and taking care of oneself for people with type 2 diabetes.

Decision: The Significance of a Reasonable Eating regimen

In the excursion of overseeing and flourishing with type 2 diabetes, the meaning of a reasonable eating regimen couldn't possibly be more significant. This cookbook has planned to give an exhaustive manual for people with type 2 diabetes, enabling them to settle on educated and good food decisions without forfeiting flavor and pleasure.

All through the parts, we've investigated different recipes and feast thoughts customized to suit the dietary necessities of those living with type 2 diabetes. From good morning meals to fulfilling primary courses, reviving refreshments to scrumptious sweets, and, surprisingly, exceptional event recipes, the cookbook has strived to offer a different scope of culinary choices to suit various preferences and inclinations.

Appreciating Flavorful Feasts with Type 2 Diabetes

It is urgent to perceive that living with type 2 diabetes doesn't mean forfeiting the joy of scrumptious feasts. By settling on careful fixing decisions, zeroing in on segment control, and embracing different healthy and supplement rich food varieties, people can deal with their glucose levels actually as well as appreciate the delight of eating.

This cookbook fills in as an important asset and a sidekick on the excursion to better wellbeing and prosperity. It is our expectation that the recipes, dinner arranging guides, and tips gave inside these pages will rouse you to make and appreciate feeding, tasty, and fulfilling feasts that advance ideal wellbeing and imperativeness.

Recall that overseeing type 2 diabetes is certainly not a single undertaking. It includes an organization with medical services professionals, the help of friends and family, and a pledge to taking care of oneself. With the right information and apparatuses, people with type 2 diabetes can lead satisfying lives, relishing every feast as a potential chance to sustain the body and support the spirit.

Determination: The Significance of a Fair Eating regimen

All things considered, we have dove into the basic meaning of keeping a decent eating regimen while living with type 2 diabetes. This cookbook has been created determined to offer an exhaustive manual for people with type 2 diabetes, enabling them to settle on educated and good food decisions without settling for less on taste and delight.

All through its pages, we have investigated a wide exhibit of recipes and feast thoughts mindfully organized to line up with the dietary necessities of those overseeing type 2 diabetes. From generous morning meals to satisfying fundamental courses, invigorating drinks to delicious sweets, and, surprisingly, unique event recipes, this cookbook has looked to introduce a different range of culinary choices to take special care of various palates and inclinations.

Getting a charge out of Delectable Dinners with Type 2 Diabetes

It is basic to recognize that existence with type 2 diabetes shouldn't compare to a relinquishment of the delight got from enjoying delicious feasts. By taking on sensible fixing choices, zeroing in on segment control, and embracing a scope of supporting, supplement rich food varieties, people can really direct their glucose levels as well as loll in the joys of gastronomy.

This cookbook tries to act as an important asset and a confided in partner in your quest for further developed wellbeing and generally prosperity. We trust that the recipes, feast arranging bits of knowledge, and useful hints found inside these pages will arouse your culinary creative mind, enabling you to specialty and relish healthy, flavorsome, and satisfying dishes that champion your wellbeing.

It is vital to perceive that the administration of type 2 diabetes is certainly not a single endeavor. It requires a cooperative relationship with medical services professionals, the consolation and backing of friends and family, and an enduring obligation to taking care of oneself. With the right information and apparatuses available to you, people living with type 2 diabetes can have improved existences, praising every feast as a valuable chance to support both body and soul.

Taking everything into account, we ask you to embrace the excursion of overseeing type 2 diabetes with good faith, tirelessness, and an appreciation for healthy, wonderful cooking. May this cookbook stand as your dependable friend, directing you in settling on edified decisions and delighting in the inclinations of a decent eating regimen fastidiously adjusted to your unmistakable prerequisites. Here's to your prosperity and the enjoyment of relishing life's culinary fortunes, each feast in turn.

Supplements

Notwithstanding the culinary excursion investigated in the first parts, this cookbook likewise gives a progression of important supplements to additionally improve your culinary experience and understanding. These addendums include:

Glossary of Cooking Terms: An extensive rundown of cooking terms and definitions to support understanding and excelling at cooking.

Rundown of Normal Fixings: A convenient reference list of ordinarily involved fixings in the recipes highlighted all through the cookbook.

Assets for Additional Data: An arranged rundown of legitimate sources and associations where you can track down extra data, direction, and backing for overseeing type 2 diabetes and keeping a solid way of life.

Record: A definite file that permits you to effectively find explicit recipes, dinner arranging tips, and other substance inside the cookbook.

With these indeces, we mean to furnish you with the instruments and information important to certainly explore the universe of cooking, settle on informed fixing decisions, and access extra assets to help your excursion towards ideal wellbeing and culinary fulfillment.